A DOCTOR OF OUR TIMES

ELLIOTT MERCER

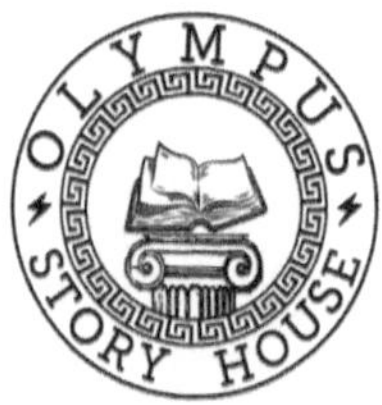

Olympus Story House

Contents

Prologue
Chapter 1 ....Nolan
Chapter 2 .... New Orleans
Chapter 3 .... Sarah
Chapter 4 .... Thoracic Surgery
Chapter 5 .... Nolan and Sarah
Chapter 6 .... Transition
Chapter 7 .... Chicago
Chapter 8 ....Sarah, Reflecting
Chapter 9 .... Chicago 2
Chapter 10 .... Financial Opportunity
Chapter 11 .... Nolan
Chapter 12 .... Nolan and Sarah, Revisited
Chapter 13 ....The Storm
Chapter 14 .... Aftermath
Chapter 15 .... Cyclone
Chapter 16 .... Debbie
Chapter 17 .... Counseling
Chapter 18 ....Money and the Practice of Medicine
Chapter 19 .... Debbie, with Demands
Chapter 20 .... Sarah, Decisive
Chapter 21 .... Young James
Chapter 22 .... Nolan, at a Crossroad
Chapter 23 ....Reinvigoration
Chapter 24 ....The Proposal
Chapter 25 .... Going Forward
Chapter 26 .... Finale
Conclusion

Prologue

NOLAN HAD WANTED TO BECOME A PHYSICIAN FOR AS LONG AS he could remember. He recalled how fascinated he'd been when his physician uncle had taken out his stethoscope and showed him how to listen for his own heartbeat; how he'd giggled when his uncle had tapped his flexed knee and got a reflex jerk of leg straightening; and how cool it was to look into his uncle's open mouth and see "that funny-looking thing hanging down behind his tongue," which Nolan was told was the uvula.

"What does it do?" Nolan had asked.

"I don't know for sure," his uncle had said. "But I'm sure that it's good for something!"

As a teenager, Nolan read several books about doctors. The most influential by far was *Arrowsmith*, the classic work by Sinclair Lewis, which tells the story of the trials and travails of a Midwestern physician. Little did young Nolan realize that some of these travails were harbingers of his own career. Years later, when his life had not turned out as he had expected it would, Nolan would reflect on his career and how, when, and why it had gone astray.

Nolan wasn't always like he had come to be, with all the money; the toys (Porsche roadster, Mercedes-Benz); the large home on the lakefront; and—oh, yes—the "other" female companions; and even his friends, so similar to him in their materialistic ways. Why? When had it all begun? Nolan didn't know for sure, since it was insidious, creeping into his life, like an infection, without warning. He'd tried on numerous occasions to figure out the *why,* even asking friends, "What happened to me? Did any of you see this happening but didn't tell me what you saw?"

Most people, like Nolan himself, at some time in their lives, have gone through the thought process, trying to make sense of what has happened and why. Because the mind is such a complicated web of intricate neurons, interwoven with such delicacy and unknowns, it may be virtually impossible to understand, much less resolve those questions. Whenever Nolan made the attempt— and he had on many occasions—the resulting outcome was mixed at best. Lying in bed at night, often with a woman at his side, had been the most common theater. Sometimes during the day, even in the midst of surgery, he'd found his mind wandering in search of answers to questions he hadn't even contemplated.

The *when* part of the questions was a little easier to figure out. Nolan could easily reflect, reconstructing where he was when he first began thinking about how much money he might be able to earn in private practice in, say, New York City or Los Angeles. It was easy to remember where he was when he went after a girl at a bar while he was already committed to another one. And Nolan could easily recall where he was when he listened to a group of physicians bragging about a new economic venture and how to profit even more from the practice of medicine.

Sometimes, the questions were clear. But how could Nolan explain how he'd gotten to where he was? What had happened over the course of the years to change him so dramatically? Did Nolan even realize that many of his friends and family couldn't recognize him as the "committed physician" they'd known and admired so long ago? Did Nolan expect and desire that he would remain this way, that he would completely separate himself from his earlier commitments?After all, Nolan had gone into medicine expecting to make a difference in the lives of others. Would those "others" turn out to be economic opportunists, rather than the ill, the disadvantaged—all those people who might benefit from his expertise?

The answers to those questions require a detailed look into Nolan's past.

CHAPTER 1
Nolan

THE VIEW FROM HIS APARTMENT WAS MAGNIFICENT. NESTLED high on Mount Sutro above the city of San Francisco, Nolan could see the Bay and the Marin County side of the Golden Gate Bridge from his porch, South San Francisco and the airport activity to his right, and Golden Gate Park directly in front. The year was 1981, and Nolan was a second-year medical school student. The medical center was just down the hill from his apartment, a short ride on his Vespa or even a reasonable walk on those days when the weather and his busy schedule would permit.

Sheer luck had found the apartment, which was actually discovered by his old high school buddy Tom, who had just taken a job with a small start-up computer firm in Silicon Valley. Tom needed a roommate to share the expenses. It wasn't cheap at the time— $1,750 per month, unfurnished, and barely within his range—but when he'd stood there for the first time last August, just before the beginning of the fall term, Nolan was hooked.

It didn't hurt that Tom and his friends all raved about the location and what a great place it was to bring women back for drinks and whatever might follow.

"This one is a can't-miss opportunity, Nolan!" pleaded Tom.

It was an easy sale.

The school year had started well. Courses in physiology, pathology, and pharmacology had replaced last year's gross anatomy and its dissections and the lab stench.

Nolan remembered his pediatrician father telling him that his copy of *Gray's Anatomy,* the bible for beginning medical students, reeked of formaldehyde for fifteen years, until his wife, Nolan's mother, threw it away.

"The aroma of that book has stayed with me for decades," Dad had related to Nolan on many occasions.

And Nolan was really enjoying the course in physical diagnosis, which included the methods of taking a patient's history and performing a physical examination. It was the first time Nolan had ever laid a hand on a person for the purpose of assessment—which organs could be palpated, how far joints could be flexed and extended, what one actually could see by looking in someone's throat. It didn't hurt that his group's patient/ model (hired by the school for educational purposes) was an attractive young woman who wasn't bothered by being seen almost naked and examined by a bunch of young (mostly) men. She seemed to enjoy the process! Of course, all this was supervised by a professor and performed professionally, but that didn't stop Nolan and his buddies from admiring the "patient's" body.

"If it hadn't been in a classroom, I would have asked her to meet me for a drink after class," said one. Still, the entire experience further reinforced Nolan's satisfaction that he was pursuing the right course in life. Nolan would become a physician, likely a surgeon, just as he had been planning for years.

Truthfully, getting into medical school had not been that difficult for him. Nolan had always excelled in the sciences in school. He was used to competition, both in the classroom and on the athletic field —he was a very capable football player (though too slow to compete in college) and a golfer who competed avidly in high school with his father, brother, and numerous friends. Nolan even played a passable flamenco guitar, which he took to Spain after two years of undergraduate college, playing in pickup bars in exchange for drinks and tips. That same guitar occupied a prominent place in the living room of his apartment for years, and he would often pick it up, primarily to entertain friends—or better yet a date—with his prowess.

With all that going for him, one might conclude that Nolan would be successful in whatever he chose to do. And they would have been right. There was that one problem, however, one that very few people (certainly not his friends or teachers) knew of—a gnawing lack of self- confidence. Nolan knew it and had tried his best to either ignore or suppress it, but that didn't always work. Its origin— who knew for sure? Was it due to his mother, who could be overbearing, often demanding, and usually not satisfied with anything he did? Like coming home from school with a report card including A-minuses or, God forbid, B-pluses? That would really set her off.

"I know that you are capable of getting straight As, Nolan. Why are you not applying yourself?"

As Nolan grew older, in his later teen years, he found himself avoiding any conversations with his mother that might provoke her and start an argument.

Or maybe his lack of confidence was related to his relationships with his siblings. Mary and Roger, each older than Nolan, each took turns in picking on him, whether on the backyard basketball court, while playing games in the house, or in the family car on long rides. There was nothing unusual about those interactions among siblings, except that his parents, Nolan had thought at the time, rarely came to his rescue. Usually, his mother would say something to the effect of, "Deal with it. It's part of growing up." No support would ever come from Mom, and his Dad ignored those situations, Nolan later realized.

That same lack of confidence also became apparent during his early dating years. Girls thought Nolan handsome, with a winning smile and a good personality. Nonetheless, he suffered from shyness and difficulty in coming up with the right words when girls were around him, unless his buddies were there to pick up the slack. And Nolan's first sexual forays, though modest in degree, were met with a hesitation that confused him. Did the girl really want him to stop kissing her? Or was it part of the expected first-attempt resistance? If only his sister or a more sympathetic, understanding woman was around to give him guidance.

Nolan's sister, Mary, understood the ambivalence that high school girls felt about romantic encounters. When he told her about one girl or another that he liked, her retort sometimes was, "Well, she obviously likes you and wants you to make a move on her. What's stopping you?" But try as he might, Nolan always stopped whenever the girl voiced the least bit of resistance.

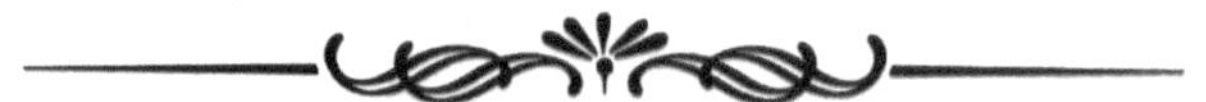

In spite of the rigors of medical school, Nolan and his buddies still found some time for fun. Golden Gate Park offered almost unlimited opportunities, even though the concerts of the 1960s—which had offered, free of charge, a chance to see legendary rock groups such as the Mamas and the Papas, Country Joe and the Fish, and Buffalo Springfield—were a thing of the past.

Later on, Nolan often said, "When I got older and had to pay to attend rock concerts, I couldn't believe that so many people had seen some of those superstars for free in San Francisco!"

And there were athletic fields in the park available for pickup soccer and softball games. Sometimes, the medical center staff participated. Just the beauty of the park, particularly in springtime, gave everyone a taste of what life could be like when one took time to smell the flowers—and more. There was also the scent of marijuana about when cruising the Haight-Ashbury district of San Francisco, formerly hippie haven. Nolan would conjecture, *I could get high just by walking around here.*

The Haight had been (and remained) an anachronism, even in liberal San Francisco. Nestled between Noe Valley and Mount Parnassus (site of the medical center), with Golden Gate Park to the north and the suburban, lily-white middle-class Sunset District to the west, the Haight stubbornly refused to succumb to the norms of city life. By the time Nolan was living close by on Mount Sutro, the Haight had changed from the freewheeling sixties. Gone were most of the flower children and relatively harmless hippies and street musicians, replaced by more hardened residents. Some of them were heavy drug users and sellers. Indeed, crack cocaine was readily available to anyone who wished to buy.

The quaint shops that sold books, musical instruments and records, and avant-garde clothing, along with the innumerable coffee shops and ethnic restaurants, were having a tough time surviving. Tourists, the heart of the economic activity during the sixties, were scared away by the drug culture.

In spite of that, the Haight, changed as it was, did survive. Many local residents and visitors continued to be attracted to the weird, unusual, and strikingly flamboyant nature of this segment of San Francisco life.

Nolan met Marcia at one of the coffee shops on Haight Street, quite by accident (literally, as he bumped into her while carrying his coffee to the outdoor table). She smiled somewhat patronizingly but responded to his apology with a warm, "Not to worry," and that broke the ice. A little mindless banter ensued and then selfintroductions.

Marcia said, "I'm a dental hygiene student at the medical center."

Nolan responded, "Well, I'd be happy to volunteer myself as one of your patients!" Although Nolan immediately regretted this ridiculous response, he nonetheless found the courage to ask her out for dinner, which she accepted. The romance, or so Nolan hoped, was about to begin. Marcia was tall and lean and pretty enough, but not so gorgeous as to be intimidating. She had beautiful long blond hair and sparkling eyes that could, Nolan thought, melt snow. Driving home on his Vespa, he almost hit a curb while daydreaming about her.

Nolan began planning his next date with Marcia immediately. First, he told Tom that, if he planned to be around that evening, he would appreciate it if Tom would find any reason to excuse himself early.

"No problem," said Tom, adding, "How long will it take you to get into her pants?" But then he agreed to Nolan's request. "I'll make myself scarce and not compete with you."

Nolan pretty much behaved himself. During dinner and the preplanned foray to the apartment, he and Marcia shared a drink and conversation with Tom and his girlfriend. Later on, when they were alone, Nolan also conducted himself as a gentleman. To his credit, Nolan had never been the type of guy to force himself onto a girl. He preferred to wait until the right time and for a signal to occur. That didn't happen this particular evening.

But the next time was different. Marcia invited him to her apartment in the Sunset District of San Francisco, where she lived solo. Very quickly, it became apparent that Marcia was ready for a more intimate relationship. In fact, it began shortly after the first drink, when she, very suddenly, approached him at his chair, parted his legs to press close to him, and began to unbutton her blouse.

"Am I a little too forward for you, or do you like it when a girl is the aggressive one? After all, I am a product of the sexual revolution."

"I can get used to it."

Most of the rest was a blur. What he remembered—and reremembered for days afterward—was how Marcia had insisted that Nolan undress her slowly, while she simultaneously reached into his pants and found his penis, which, of course, had become very hard, very quickly. Marcia turned out to be a little quirky in her sexual desires—more so than his previous partners. But Nolan was entranced, allowing her to guide him through the entire highintensity act at her (sometimes breathless) pace.

The relationship continued for several weeks, interrupted only by their prerequisite classes, studies, and exams. It would be an understatement, however, to say that Nolan was enjoying himself or that he truly was smitten with her. Daydreaming, night dreaming, and all manner of mental images and gymnastics were the results of their vigorous sexual relationship.

The end was as sudden as the beginning. Marcia stated starkly and without warning that she had become bored, and she made it quite clear that she wished to move on.

"But I really like you, Marcia! Why do you suddenly want to break it off?"

"I'm just not ready for a commitment right now, Nolan. Truthfully, I just don't think that you're the right guy for me, and it's easier to do this now than to wait for who knows what."

Nolan struggled to maintain his emotions and self-control but finally gathered himself together and told Marcia, "OK, I'm out of here forever."

It was over. When Nolan left her apartment for what would prove to be the last time, he felt an ache, a loss unlike anything he had ever experienced. That feeling would stay with Nolan and influence his future relationships for quite some time.

When the second school year had ended, Nolan began the clinical phase of medical school. This marked a dramatic change, the beginning of a more thorough interaction with patients, both on hospital wards and in the clinical environment.

For Nolan and his colleagues, that meant rotating on monthly medical services—orthopedics, pediatrics, obstetrics and gynecology, and internal medicine, along with the area to which he most looked forward, surgery. As it happened, strictly by circumstance, he began with obstetrics and gynecology at San Francisco General Hospital, SFGH or "the General," as it was fondly (sometimes not so fondly) referred to by staff, nurses, and patients. Many of them had been participants in medical activity at the General for years.

SFGH was originally built in 1872 in the Mission District of San Francisco, then, as now, home to many of the indigent, lessfortunate residents of the city. The original wooden structure was destroyed by the 1906 earthquake, and the hospital was rebuilt in the brick Italian Renaissance style, completed in 1915. It remained as such into the twenty-first century. Essentially operating as a public hospital, it served a large segment of San Francisco's indigent population and served as a teaching hospital for medical students, residents, and nurses. It also became a renowned clinical research center under the University of California at San Francisco (UCSF) umbrella.

The stories involving the hospital were legion. Many trauma victims had ended up at SFGH over the decades. As well, the down-and-out of the city, often drug- and/ or alcohol-suffused, were attended to in its emergency room when the need arose, which it did frequently. The underground hospital tunnels, built to connect the vast separated buildings, saw assaults, drug dealing, dog races, and all manner of nefarious activities over the years.

In 1967, the classic movie *Bullitt,* starring Steve McQueen and Robert Vaughn, was partially filmed in those tunnels, which were previously poorly illuminated but were upgraded by the producers for filming purposes. Those upgrades became a functioning part of the hospital. Some of the scenes required filming in an intensive care unit (ICU). Filming obviously couldn't take place during real-time hospital activity, so the hospital administration told the film company that it would have to construct an "imitation" ICU, staffed with actors as patients and medical personnel. That happened, and subsequently, when the filming was complete, the fully equipped ICU was turned over to the hospital, ready for use. *The San Francisco Chronicle* heralded that action as one of the best examples of private/public partnership in the city's history.

It was in that institution that Nolan Burkett first began his clinical clerkship as a third-year medical student. His first monthlong rotation began on the ob-gyn service. On Nolan's very first day, he found himself in the delivery room area, attending a "grand multip," medical jargon for a woman who had given birth multiple times and was about to do so, rapidly, again. When she was placed on the delivery table, her feet carefully positioned in stirrups, she began to alternately moan and scream in cadence with her contractions. These were coming at increasingly close intervals, and one of the nurses, standing just over Nolan's left shoulder, said, in a manner both menacing and condescending, "Well, *Doctor,* what are you going to do now?"

Nolan answered somewhat nervously, "Well, I'm going to get ready to perform a delivery."

By the time Nolan had washed his hands thoroughly, donned his gown, and been helped into surgical gloves, there was another short scream and a burst of profanity (from either the patient or the nurse). Before he knew it, a live baby had burst forth and literally fallen into the hands of the waiting nurse. The nurse again looked at him, this time with a combination of resignation and pity. She then gave the newborn a quick slap on the back, which resulted in the first cry in the new world the infant had entered.

"Next time, Dr. Burkett," the nurse admonished, "you should get ready for the delivery a little more quickly!"

Nolan didn't know whether to clap or exhale with relief, so he did neither; rather, he determined that the next time, he would be better prepared.

Just when Nolan had begun to get the hang of it in the delivery room, the month ended, and he moved on to an orthopedic surgery rotation. Orthopedics (*ortho* to the medical staff) in the 1980s was a far cry from the modern-day practice, which now involves such complex surgical procedures as joint replacements and spinal fusions. At that time, it mostly consisted of dealing with trauma, the associated skeletal fractures, and the resultant repairs that followed. Nolan spent entire days in the casting room, with its plaster of paris casts, splints, and vast assortment of bandages utilized for virtually every part of the human body. Nolan became quite facile with their applications, to the point where the ortho technicians (who did most of this work, thereby freeing the staff for the more illustrious surgical procedures) gave him pretty much free rein to work with minimal supervision.

"Hey, Doc, you all ready with that cast? This patient will be all healed up before you get that thing on his arm!"

Both Nolan and the technician laughed and continued casting and bandaging through the night. Nolan enjoyed the rotation and the banter with colleagues and the techs. He quickly decided, however, that this was not on his career list; Nolan felt that boredom would set in quite quickly. He had not had an opportunity to learn about the more sophisticated aspects of orthopedics.[1]

Pediatrics was a different matter. For this, Nolan moved to the UCSF university hospital on Parnassus Avenue, close to his apartment. Here he spent a most satisfying month. Although much of the work was mundane, involving well-baby checkups, immunizations, and routine infectious disease care of mostly notvery- ill children (and their anxious parents), there was another side to it. That involved attending to those unfortunate children who suffered from cancers, such as leukemia, Wilms' kidney tumors, and lymphomas. Nolan attended on the cancer service of the hospital for two weeks.

One of Nolan's patients was an eleven-year-old boy who had had his leg amputated for osteogenic sarcoma, an often fatal bone cancer that had recurred, with metastases now in his lungs. One day on rounds when Nolan entered the boy's room, the boy, with his parents by the bedside, proudly showed Nolan his new baseball glove.

"When I get out of the hospital," the boy said to Nolan with a big smile, "I'm going to get a new leg and become a baseball player!"

Nolan left the room shortly after in tears, thinking, *I'll remember his smile and his excitement over his baseball glove for the rest of my life.*

Pediatrics was Nolan's father's specialty. And for a while, Nolan considered what it might be like to become a pediatrician and join his father in practice. He was never quite sure why he decided against doing that; of course, it would have been convenient to go into practice with his father after the completion of a residency. But idealism was a strong characteristic of Nolan's at that time, and he didn't want to take the easy path for the wrong reasons.

Would I really choose to be a pediatrician if my father wasn't one?

The Oedipus complex, which is used to describe the subliminal sexual ambivalence of a male child toward his mother, has a somewhat similar psychological dilemma involving a male child and his father. Oft-times it surfaces as jealousy and a competitive attitude between the two. It is not possible to know if that problem existed between Nolan and his father. But Nolan did resent that his father rarely took a personal interest in whatever he was thinking or doing at any particular time.

And, Nolan knew that the father/son relationship could well be strained in a professional partnership. He told his roommate, "I just don't know if I can spend my career working alongside my father. We didn't spend that much time together when I was growing up, so I don't know how I would handle it now."

Nolan struck pediatrics from his career choices list.

The general surgery rotation was, predictably, his favorite. He was able to extend his time on that service by an additional month by using a portion of his elective time, thereby giving him almost nine weeks of continuous participation with the SFGH surgical team. As a student, he wouldn't perform even the most basic of surgical procedures, such as herniorrhaphies and appendectomies. But in the emergency room, where life-threatening events took place almost daily—especially on weekend nights, when the infamous "knife and gun clubs," ubiquitous to cities like San Francisco, turned out patients like a water spigot—it was all-hands-on-deck. Nolan sutured severe lacerations, affixed temporary splints to major fractures, and even probed knife wounds to the chest and abdomen to determine whether or not prompt surgical exploration was required.

One of the senior surgical residents with whom he had bonded early on was fond of saying repeatedly, "It's a fucking madhouse out there!"

On one evening, a fourteen-year-old boy was brought in to the ER by ambulance and whisked into the emergency bay, with blood gushing from his groin, the result of a knife wound. There was blood everywhere, and when nurses and doctors frantically assessed him and tried to obtain his vital signs, his blood pressure barely registered. Shortly after, the boy's heart stopped, and in spite of CPR and a simultaneous race to the operating room, he died. For weeks afterward, Nolan questioned himself—was there anything more that he could have done to save that poor boy's life? If he had immediately clamped down on the wound, could he have stopped the flow of blood?

"Maybe if I had been a little quicker, if I had been there to compress his groin and stop the bleeding a little earlier, he would be alive now," Nolan said to one of his colleagues upon learning of the boy's death.

The residents, seeing his pain and self-doubt, assured him that nothing that he or anyone else could have done would have saved the boy. But Nolan was unsure whether that was really true.

Other patients fared better, and Nolan gained confidence in his ability to make a difference. He developed pride in his suturing skills, admiring some of his facial repair work to the extent that he thought about possibly becoming a plastic surgeon. That feeling was amplified when he rotated through the surgical burn unit, a very highly regarded service at SFGH. The cosmetic repairs of severe burns, performed by highly skilled doctors, was impressive. People severely disfigured by burns were miraculously returned to at least a reasonable appearance, to the extent that they were no longer the objects of dispassionate stares. *I always marveled at the incredible efforts and the successes of the burn unit team, and strongly considered doing a fellowship in burn repair, following a surgical residency.*

In the operating room, a medical student such as Nolan was usually relegated to the role of surgical retraction—that is, holding a spoon-like or curved stainless steel instrument for many minutes or even hours against the inside of a body cavity, thus allowing the surgeon to see the region of interest and enabling him or her to perform the task at hand.

Retraction was tedious and somewhat demanding work. If one relaxed and/or moved the retractor without being asked to do so by the surgeon, the result was often a severe reprimand, possibly even replacement by another student, resident, or—heaven forbid—a surgical nurse. Many of those nurses, like Nolan's obstetrical nurse mentioned earlier, held little regard for medical students. Some of them believed, often with justification, that they, the nurses, were more valuable in the operating room than the students. Nolan and his classmates took great pains to see that that did not happen.

The end of a long day in the operating room was completed with *rounds*—evaluating each patient with the residents and nurses; performing minor tasks, such as bandage changes and blood draws for the laboratory; and determining how well (or poorly, in some cases) each patient was doing. Following that, there was the workup of the newly admitted patients, which had to be completed before the end of the day or night so that the attending residents and staff could make the requisite decisions during morning rounds. If one was really lucky, he or she would finish these labors by midnight and grab a few hours' sleep in either the hospital's on-call room or, if truly fortunate, at home.

Nolan often stated to no one in particular, "I've never been so exhausted in my life!"

The surgical services were generally regarded— by students, interns, and residents alike—as the most physically demanding of all the medical school rotations. Regardless, Nolan was smitten with surgery, and reaffirmed his commitment to become a surgeon.

In June 1981, the US Centers for Disease Control (CDC) published an article titled "Pneumocystis carinii Pneumonia (PCP)," identifying five gay men in Los Angeles who were found to be infected with a then-unknown virus. Two had died by the time the article was published in the prestigious *New England Journal of Medicine*. This virus later became known as the Acquired Immunodeficiency Syndrome, or AIDS, and would rapidly become a scourge in the United States and throughout the world.

When Nolan began his first rotation in internal medicine in spring 1983, the AIDS epidemic was in full swing.

Particularly in urban, socioeconomically disadvantaged cities such as San Francisco, there existed a large contingent of homosexual males who were becoming infected and dying at alarming rates. The fact that heterosexual persons who'd had blood transfusions within the last several years also became infected did not receive the attention of most of the public. And many political leaders, including the then president of the United States, had precious little sympathy for affected homosexuals.

The pharmaceutical industry had little incentive or interest in developing therapeutic medication or vaccinations for AIDS in the early days of the epidemic. Most AIDS-related care was supportive, and that resulted in an extremely high death rate for those who became infected. Ironically, a significant number of people developed AIDS as a result of blood transfusion contamination; that fact was unknown to the majority of people, however, who generally accepted that the disease occurred solely among homosexuals.

San Francisco Medical Center established the world's first dedicated outpatient AIDS clinic in January 1983. Fortuitously, this was where Nolan and several of his classmates were assigned. Prior to the AIDS epidemic, a rotation in internal medicine mainly revolved around caring for patients with the more usual afflictions—diabetes; hypertension; and infections such as staphylococcus, streptococcus, and a whole host of other maladies. Some of them were quite rare and very interesting to a medical student—scleroderma (a disfiguring and mysterious disease primarily of the skin) or endocrine disorders, such as hyperthyroidism and pituitary gland dysfunctions. And there were the ubiquitous but all-too-common cancers, many of which were uncurable but required significant therapeutic measures. The medical students continued to be involved with patients who suffered from these and other illnesses, but it was AIDS that knocked them—

and the entire medical community—for a loop. Prior to the epidemic, no one, not even the experienced staff internists, had seen or been involved in something so unusual, so depressing, and so often fatal as AIDS.

Ward 86, the outpatient unit created solely for the treatment of AIDS at SFGH, was an incredible sight. The mostly male patients were emaciated, with open and festering sores and glandular swelling that, in some, became recognized as Kaposi sarcoma, a particularly onerous cancer.

Malnutrition resulted, in part, from lesions in the mouth and throat that made eating unbearable; even swallowing a glass of water was painful. Most of the patients were itinerant and had no steady job or means of support; they relied almost entirely on community health services, which were paid by the taxpayer. This also had ramifications, as the costs were enormous, and many politicians, responding to conservative public opinion, were loath to provide funding for those patients' care.

When Nolan and his classmates, along with the attending staff— doctors, nurses, orderlies, laboratory, and X-ray technicians—spent long days and nights caring for these poor souls, their psyches alternated between depression and despair. In those early AIDS days, there were few recoveries. Even when recovery seemed to occur, it was usually temporary remission. Nolan had difficulty sleeping, even when he was totally exhausted after a grueling twelve- to sixteen-hour stint on the ward. The idealism that resulted in Nolan's venture into the medical field was severely tested, but he refused to succumb to despair. Nolan continued to perform his duties as best he could, hoping that would make a difference.

Nolan had good relationships with several members of the medical staff, including Michael Stewart, a medical school classmate who was gay. At that time, most homosexuals remained "in the closet"; broad acceptance by the public was the exception rather than the rule. Michael, however, was always comfortable in his own skin. At social gatherings and parties, Michael was often in the company of another male, and it became obvious that this was by design. None of his classmates seemed bothered by it, or if they were, they kept it to themselves.

I used to joke with Michael about the good-looking girls and guys at our medical class parties. Michael always laughed and talked as if it was just normal banter. Later in my life, I realized how insensitive I'd been, how clueless to the ambiguities and ambivalences that a gay person experienced. It was only after I saw the devastation that AIDS brought on—the heartbreak between couples, family members, and friends—that I realized how naive and clueless I was.

There likely were other gay people in Nolan's class, but Nolan knew only Michael well; they had been first-year partners in the gross anatomy dissection class. Even though Nolan and Michael didn't attend on the same service on Ward 86, they had frequent contact in school and social gatherings. It was during those times that Nolan attempted, carefully at first, to ask Michael, not so much about homosexual behavior—that would have been too intrusive—but how he felt about his own safety. Most gay men knew the risks, Nolan realized, but did they consciously consider that before sexual contact? Or were they so driven by their sexuality that they were willing to accept the consequences of AIDS?

During the later phase of his medical education, Nolan had tried his level best to understand. It wasn't easy, and he knew that Michael knew that Nolan would never be able to fully comprehend what Michael and his friends were thinking about AIDS. The most that Nolan could expect of himself was to not prejudge homosexuality in general and his patient in particular. *I was determined to provide the best care that I could for the AIDS patients and to accept their lifestyle, regardless of the horrors of the disease.*

What happened was often tragic. So many men (rarely a woman in the early AIDS days) were affected, and the medical care remained primarily palliative. The nursing staff was far more accomplished at tending to the needs of most of the patients; doctors always shied away from the intimacies of personal care, and Nolan was no exception. Nolan would find almost any excuse to leave the bedside when a patient had soiled himself or needed assistance getting to the bathroom.

There were some positive moments. One young man, who seemed doomed from the moment he entered the hospital, made an amazing recovery. Nolan grew fond of Jamie, frequently spending his lunch hour with him and often wheeling Jamie onto the patio for some sunshine and fresh air. They discussed a wide range of topics. Jamie was an accomplished artist, talented enough to have some of his watercolors shown at the San Francisco Museum of Art in Golden Gate Park.

"Jamie, I would love to see some of your work on display. Will you let me know when we can do that together? When you're discharged from the hospital, the two of us will visit the museum."

"Sure, Doc, as soon as I get out of this hellhole, we'll get together —I promise."

That never came to pass. After Jamie left the hospital, the two of them never saw each other again.

Another medical event involving Nolan occurred when a patient on the ward suddenly became hypotensive and collapsed on the floor. Examination revealed an acute abdomen, meaning abdominal pain, severe tenderness to palpation, and what seemed to indicate to the surgical resident summoned internal bleeding. The patient (Nolan didn't know his name at the time) was rushed to the operating room. Nolan, with his mental fixation on surgery, talked his way into the OR and assisted with the abdominal exploration. The surgeon immediately recognized that the patient's spleen had ruptured, resulting in an abdominal cavity filled with blood. Heroic efforts resulted in the patient surviving the operation and eventually returning to Ward 86. He remained there past the time that Nolan rotated onto another service.

It was a long month for Nolan. But the result was an appreciation for the incredibly talented and committed medical staff—the nurses, the doctors, and all manner of personnel—that attended to those critically ill patients. When he next rotated on an internal medicine service at the university hospital, it was as if he was on an extended vacation. The stresses on that and other similar services were minor by comparison to what he had experienced on Ward 86.2

The rest of the third and fourth years of medical school went by in a blur. Other rotations in pediatrics, neurology, and cardiac surgery took place. Nolan and his schoolmates made it through with the usual combination of effort, some sleepless nights, and fatigue, which was the usual fare for medical students. Then there were the final exams, ending with the state board of medicine examination, a requirement for licensure as a physician. Nolan and his classmates worried constantly about the board exam.

Shortly following the exam, Nolan and his friend Paul were celebrating over a pizza dinner. They each marveled at how concerned they had been. Nolan said to Paul, "I sweated bullets worrying about the board examination. I thought there was no way I would pass. I hadn't had any time to study for the exam, what with the demands of the rotations. When I was notified that I had passed the exam, I was convinced that the examiners hadn't really reviewed my answers!"

Nolan knew of no one in his class who didn't pass the exam.

By the time of graduation—a momentous affair that his parents and siblings, a couple of aunts and uncles, and a few close friends attended—even his mother showed excitement and pride in her son's accomplishments, telling others, "I always knew that Nolan could do it, and now he's proven me right!"

Nolan, later hearing of his mother's comment, said to his sister, "Mom, in her inevitable way, continues to take credit for every good thing that I've ever done. Nothing will ever change her behavior, I'm convinced."

"In her own way, Mom is proud of you, Nolan; she just doesn't know how to express that."

Nolan's pediatrician father was more taciturn but was obviously thrilled that Nolan was now a doctor. Nolan never determined whether or not his father had anticipated that Nolan would decide to join him in his pediatrics practice, but it was time for Nolan to move on.

Nolan had chosen and been accepted for an internship/surgical residency program at Charity Hospital in New Orleans. Following graduation, Nolan had one week to pack his possessions and load them into his Honda Accord; sell his Vespa; give away countless items, including his precious but rarely used surfboard; and make the "goodbye rounds" to his friends and classmates, most of whom he would never see again. In later years, Nolan would muse about how much those medical school days had meant to him and about those friendships that he had established but often taken for granted. He thought back countless times to all the fun that his classmates and he had had, in spite of the stresses of medical school. *Those were, without doubt, the best days of my life. I'd gladly relive them, if only I could.*

CHAPTER 2
New Orleans

CHARITY HOSPITAL, OWNED AND OPERATED BY LOUISIANA State University, best known as LSU (the Tigers of fabled college football fame), was founded in 1736 with an endowment from a French shipbuilder. From its inception and continuing as a rebuilt hospital following its severe destruction by Hurricane Katrina, Charity Hospital provided medical care for any Louisiana resident who could not afford to pay. As the hospital was situated in the heart of the city, virtually everyone who lived in New Orleans had occasion either to become a patient in the hospital or to work nearby, often on its very grounds.

Nolan chose LSU/Charity primarily because of its renowned surgical training program. It was particularly renowned in the subspecialty of thoracic surgery. As in most public hospitals that served a large urban, primarily indigent population, thousands of surgical procedures were performed.

Many of those were related to trauma, and for thoracic surgery in particular, that offered opportunities for Nolan and other residents to become hands-on surgeons early in training. That occurred rarely in many highly academic university training programs, which often did not have the number of cases to allow for younger residents to operate.

One of SFGH's staff physicians, a Dr. Thomas Charlton, had trained at Charity and was influential in Nolan's decision to apply. Dr. Charlton also provided a very strong recommendation to LSU's residency search committee. So when Nolan was matched with Charity by the national medical residency program, his number one choice (SFGH was number two), it was no surprise to him.

Dr. Charlton told Nolan, "By the time that you finish your surgical training at Charity, you'll be confident and be ready to practice surgery anywhere in the world. In fact, I hope that when that happens, you'll consider coming back to SFGH as a staff physician."

Nolan was flattered by the words and immediately filed them in his memory bank for future consideration. *Too early to begin to think about the future, though, he thought, with at least five years' training ahead of him.*

Nolan knew precious little about the South, in general, or New Orleans, in particular. He had attended Mardi Gras as a college sophomore, but that involved mostly liquor-lubricated days and nights in the Bourbon Street region, some raucous parades, and a ton of music—the jazz bands on the streets and in the bars and hundreds of unusually garbed people playing instruments, washboards, and tin can drums on street corners. By the time he dragged himself back to college from that sojourn, he was a total wreck; it took over a week for him to recover and to get his mind and body back into gear. He had minimal recollection of anything related to New Orleans.

Later he mused, *I'm glad I got that out of my system. Don't think that I could survive for very long at that pace. Five hours of sleep in five days just won't cut it.*

Nolan's entire knowledge base for Southern culture, politics, and history came from three books he had read—*The Sound and the Fury* by William Faulkner, a classic novel depicting a dysfunctional family and dystopic racism; Robert Penn Warren's Nobel Prize-winning *All the King's Men,* primarily detailing the Huey Long dynasty and hard-nosed Louisiana politics; and *Huckleberry Finn,* Mark Twain's masterpiece. Anything else pertaining to the South, including its culture, long-standing poverty, and persistent racism, were not on his mind at that time. Even the history of the civil rights movement in the South had little impact on Nolan. He had long ago put Martin Luther King and his efforts aside, focusing entirely on his surgical training program, which was about to begin.

Nolan made it through a not-so-leisurely five-day cross-country drive to New Orleans. He would have liked to have stopped at some beautiful and interesting places along the way. But he chose to drive past Zion and Bryce National Parks and sped through the rolling hills of West Texas. Time was of the essence. Nolan had not arranged for living quarters in New Orleans, and he knew no one there (none of his classmates or other residents, as far as he knew, had chosen Charity Hospital for their advanced training).

Upon arrival in New Orleans, Nolan went to an LSU-run voluntary placement center and found a nice apartment on Perdido Street, only six blocks from the hospital. It was a relatively new apartment complex that had good security and functioning air-conditioning (a must in hot, humid New Orleans), so he grabbed it. Real estate was much less costly than in San Francisco, so Nolan could afford to room solo.

I've had enough of living with others—having to wade through their strewn clothes and finding dirty dishes stacked in the kitchen and sometimes even strange people sleeping on the living room sofa. I'll be married to my next roommate!

On the same day he moved in, he noticed an attractive blond woman enter the apartment complex and go up the stairs, presumably to her apartment. Nolan momentarily considered following her and saying hello but decided against it. There would likely be a better time. So for the next two days, he explored the city. Being located only a couple of blocks from famed Canal Street and the French Quarter, Nolan sought out many of the famous spots he'd not seen on his previous trip—the historic Saint James African Methodist Church; Preservation Hall and its jazz museum; restaurants such as Antoine's and Brennan's (where he knew he couldn't afford to dine); and Woldenberg Park, along the banks of the Mississippi River.

On his following day, exhausted from his long drive and from moving into the apartment, Nolan collapsed onto his blow-up bed (no furniture as yet) to sleep and woke later to prepare for the beginning of a six-year stint at LSU Medical Center.

Nolan started with a flourish. Medical school and SFGH had prepared him very well for the surgical residency program. Although, technically, he was beginning as an intern, the usual first-year role after graduation, the internship was integrated into the surgical residency program. He began on a general surgical rotation that was active, well-run, and staffed by very competent senior residents and board-certified surgeons. In addition, the surgical nurses were first class, capable of managing the most complex patients seemingly with ease. The facility was quite old, and some of the rooms and equipment were dated, but that didn't really bother him. The only real negative was that the air-conditioning was marginal, at best. With the heat of summer upon him, the days were often quite uncomfortable, especially in the operating rooms. The combination of surgical gowns and masks, along with the intense operating room lights, made it seem as if they were operating in a sauna.

Nolan said to one of the senior surgical nurses, "How do you guys survive these conditions during the summer? I feel like I need a change of clothes after five minutes in here."

She responded, "You'll get used to it after a while. And even if you don't get used to it, there really isn't much choice. Survive or succumb—that's what I've learned from my eight years working here as a nurse in the operating room."

By the end of the summer, Nolan often functioned as the first assistant, meaning that his hands were within inches of the primary surgeon's. Soon after, he was given his first opportunity to operate as the primary surgeon. Once, when beginning an emergency appendectomy, he said to an LSU medical student who was in the operating room, "We'll make the initial incision at McBurney's point— that's a point one third of the distance between the anterior-superior iliac spine and the umbilicus, the best site for locating the appendix." Nolan was beginning to function like an instructor (at least to medical students), and he enjoyed doing so.

Other operations, including herniorrhaphies (hernia repair) and cholecystectomies (gall bladder removal) followed. The more complex operations, such as gastrectomy (stomach removal) and colectomy (removal of a portion of the colon), were more involved and difficult. And for these, Nolan reverted to a lower position on the surgical team. But he was gaining useful experience, and he loved it!

One junior resident, two years Nolan's senior by training, went out of his way to befriend him, initially in the hospital but soon afterward during their occasional days off. His name was Ralph, and he was quite a guy. Born and raised in Sioux City, Iowa, the son of farmers, Ralph was married with two children. He was considerably older than Nolan. In fact, he had been a medic in the Vietnam War and was already well into his thirties when he entered medical school. A quiet, politically conservative fellow, Ralph nonetheless was a terrific storyteller. When prodded by his buddies, Ralph would talk about "the war" in a fashion that mesmerized his audience.

Ralph once told Nolan, "Helicopters evacuated injured soldiers, even civilians, daily. When they reached the field hospital, the first thing we would do was triage."

Triage is the process of separating patients into three groups—the first is those whose injuries are minor and stabilized; the second, those whose injuries are life-threatening and require immediate intervention; and the third, those for whom the only thing to be done is to alleviate their pain with narcotics and wait for them to die. Triage was an outgrowth of lessons learned by the army medical corps during World War II. In spite of the gruesome and emotionally detached nature of the process, triage has resulted in significant improvement in war-related survival statistics.

Ralph continued, "The injuries were incredible, and the suffering endured by those brave souls unimaginable. For weeks, I would lie on my cot during rest hours and wonder how people could do such unimaginable things to one another. Finally, it dawned on me that these people were merely the victims of decisions made by those of higher rank—the generals and, in particular, the politicians. The latter, of course, were nowhere to be seen on the battlefield."

Life-or-death situations were common events in Vietnam, so Ralph had been steeped in the world of surgical trauma as a medic, without having a formal medical education. "It was there that I decided," he told others, "that if I survived the war, I'd go to medical school, train to become a trauma surgeon, and give back whatever I could, in honor of my wounded or killed comrades."

Nolan felt, *I wish I could have had similar experiences, though I could certainly do without the horror of war. Some of the things Ralph has seen and done can never be duplicated in a civilian hospital setting.*

Nolan would later reflect on the first time he was invited to Ralph's home for dinner. Ralph's wife, June, and their two young children greeted and welcomed him as if he were a family member. The dinner itself was fine, but it was the warmth of the family and the home that resonated with Nolan. For the first time since he'd arrived in New Orleans, Nolan missed his own family. Simultaneously, he began to consider what it might be like to start a family himself. He knew he had quite a way to go for that. Nolan hadn't met a woman outside of the hospital, much less been on a date, since he'd arrived in New Orleans.

CHAPTER 3
Sarah

NOLAN SAW HER AGAIN ABOUT A MONTH AFTER HE HAD MOVED into the apartment. They were both taking out the garbage and met at one of the backyard trash cans. (Later on, he would remind her of that romantic first encounter.)

"I'm Nolan Burkett, and I live in that apartment across the way, directly above you."

Sarah said in reply, "Hi. I'm Sarah." (She didn't state her last name, which Nolan later thought was her being cautious.) "And I've been living here for a couple of years. Nice to meet you."

They engaged in a little bit more small talk and then said goodbye and parted ways. Nolan, however, had gained valuable information— Sarah was an ICU nurse at Tulane Medical Center, another major hospital complex in downtown New Orleans; she had no roommates (and, therefore, was most certainly single). Nolan had hesitated and hadn't thought to ask for her telephone number; or maybe he was too unsure of himself to ask.

The next time they encountered each other was in the hallway, and this time, Nolan asked her for and obtained her contact information, including her last name (Hawkins), apartment address, and phone number. He asked, somewhat abashedly, for permission to call her "soon," and she told him that that would be okay with her.

A few days later, Nolan called Sarah and arranged a coffee date at the Tulane Medical Center. She was working the night shift and slept during the day, so that was the best they could come up with. Again, a less-than-romantic encounter, but that didn't seem to matter to either of them. There seemed to be mutual interest right away—they had similar professional careers, were close in age, and there seemed to be mutual physical attraction.

Sarah was blond; this seemed to be a recurring characteristic for his female friends. She was also very attractive, with piercing blue eyes and a dimpled smile that reminded him, curiously, of his sister, Mary. In addition, Sarah spoke softly but with a confidence that was calming to Nolan. He was not intimidated by her, as he had been by some women previously.

"I've been a nurse for almost two years, following graduation from the Tulane School of Nursing. I considered but decided against leaving the city for something different. But, I'm a 'daughter of the South,' and my family lives close by. So, here I am."

"Well, I moved here for a surgical residency. This is as far away from my family as I could be and still be in the United States. I'm a fish out of water in the South, so maybe you can teach me a little bit about it."

Sarah's response was interesting to Nolan. She said, "My experience with Westerners is that they like visiting the South, particularly New Orleans, but mostly they leave and return 'home' when it becomes feasible."

Nolan sensed that Sarah would have liked to try living somewhere else, but he decided to not pursue the subject.

Nolan told her a little more about himself, mostly his excitement regarding the medical program and his satisfaction with it so far. When they parted, Nolan asked if he could see her a second time, and she responded positively.

Nolan thought, That'll keep my mind occupied outside of surgery for several days!

Their next date was more substantial. They met for a nice Cajunstyle dinner at one of Sarah's favorite restaurants, followed by a bluesy nightclub in the French Quarter.

Nolan learned that Sarah was a musician and that, like him, she had traveled abroad. She'd taken her violin with her, visiting and occasionally playing in small clubs in London and Dublin. "I loved being in Ireland. Doesn't hurt that I'm of Irish ancestry, and I even found a couple of distant relatives in Northern Ireland. They were having a tough time dealing with 'the troubles,' the ongoing violence between the Irish Catholics and Protestants. They live in Londonderry, right in the middle of it. It's very difficult, and I don't see any end in sight."

Nolan said, "Amazing! I just finished the book Trinity by Leon Uris. I was spellbound. Had no idea of the history of the conflict, that it has been going on for hundreds of years. Now because of you, I'll be able to relate to the story and to the characters."

Sarah was impressed with Nolan. *He's a very serious guy, unlike some of my previous boyfriends who spend most of their time talking about sports and themselves. She ruminated, We'll see where this goes.*

Sarah went on to talk about her family, which had been in the South since the mid-nineteenth century. Her grandfather had a thriving cotton mill near Shreveport, which her father and his siblings inherited and had subsequently owned and operated for more than seventy-five years. Their family home was next to the mill, and Sarah lived there until she left for college in the late 1970s. Sarah gave a brief description of life "on the plantation," as she called it, and Nolan could tell that not every remembrance was positive.

She and her three sisters had a nanny named Charlotte, who Sarah described as a loving black woman who had her own family. But Charlotte lived in the Hawkins' home by herself much of the time. "In the more than ten years that Charlotte and I lived together, my sisters and I never met Charlotte's husband or four children," Sarah told Nolan. "I can't believe that we let that happen."

During the early years, Sarah's upbringing and home life were quite traditional. As the second of the four Hawkins girls, she was alternately cared for and picked on by her older sister, and Sarah served in the same role for her younger sibs. Overall, they were quite close with one another and shared all their secrets, peeves, and grievances. Their mother was caring and nurturing, but, as was noticeable to all the girls, she took a back seat to their father in family matters. "Papa," as the girls called him, was a garrulous, outgoing man who obviously loved his daughters but had old-school expectations for them.

"Girls can and should get an education, but their primary goal in life is to marry and raise a family," he would say. That was how his grandparents, parents, brothers, and sisters conducted their lives, and he saw no reason to change his mind on the subject.

"Beginning in high school, I knew that I wanted to—had to—go away to school," Sarah told Nolan, "if I wanted any chance of developing my own lifestyle, without the constraints of my parents, particularly Papa. My sisters and I talked about it all the time. I was the only one who was adamant about it. My sisters were perfectly fine with continuing their education in the South and didn't really understand why I wanted to get away."

Papa James spent most of his time at the mill. At home, he preferred to spend time with his hunting dogs or in his expansive backyard. He raised a variety of vegetables and grew beautiful magnolias—rather, his hired hand Jacob tended them; James enjoyed patrolling the yard, barking orders to Jacob.

On those uncommon occasions when James engaged his daughters in serious discussions, it usually was on topics such as what they planned to do with their lives and where they planned to attend college. Unfortunately, James was more adept at offering opinions than listening to others, so Sarah never believed that her father was interested in what *she* thought, merely that she would naturally follow his advice.

Sarah was becoming more comfortable talking to Nolan—maybe the wine helped with that. She decided to tell Nolan about "one serious episode involving me and Papa. I was sixteen years old. Papa kept a small statue in the front driveway, which was a black attendant that welcomed visitors with a white-toothed grin. I told Papa one day that I found this racially demeaning. Papa exploded in rage, accusing me of 'buying into those crazy liberal ideas of civil rights organizers and eastern and California college degenerates.'"

Sarah told Nolan that her father had been raised in a stereotypical Southern family setting and that the family had owned slaves until the Civil War. She said he was totally uninterested in or willing to consider changing his attitudes regarding black people; nor would he be altering his way of life. Sarah said the encounter ended abruptly. "I was in tears." The statue remained.

When it came time for college, Sarah initially wanted to study to become a doctor. Her maternal uncle was a successful pediatrician in Baton Rouge, and Sarah adored him; she felt closer to him than she did her immediate family. No one—not Sarah, her teachers, or her family— doubted her intelligence or ability to become a doctor, but Sarah wasn't sure that she wanted to put in the years of training to get there. She said to Nolan, "Four years of undergraduate education, four years of medical school, and two to four years of residency just seemed like too much time. In addition, I always enjoyed talking with people about their emotions and difficulties, rather than studying endlessly the science courses needed to go to medical school. That may have been a cop-out, but it was how I felt at the time. So, I chose to become a nurse."

When it came time to pick a college, Sarah didn't spend time or effort to find a school far away from home, which surprised her family. They had expected she would go away to school.

"I look back and realize I was not mature enough to make that decision to leave home," she told Nolan. "I had no role models for doing so. No one in my family had ever left the South for school, and no one encouraged me to do so. I just took the easy path." "Was it the right decision?" Nolan asked.

She shook her head. "I don't know, but I do wish that I had at least considered it more seriously. I think my parents, though opposed to any of their children moving away, would have come around. I'll never know for sure."

So Sarah matriculated to nearby Tulane University; obtained her degree in literature; and, following a year's travel and living in Europe, enrolled in Tulane University Nursing School. Two years later, following graduation, she took a job as an ICU nurse with Tulane's university hospital. She was immediately placed in the medical ICU, where her patients all were critically ill—their illnesses running the gamut from complications of strokes to uncontrolled diabetes to hypertension to metastatic cancer.

Sarah said, "It was stressful and hard work, but I felt that I was needed and appreciated, even by the attending physicians, who sometimes take nurses for granted. At least in the ICU, the doctors voiced their appreciation and admiration for what we nurses did for the patients and in particular, their worried families."

Sarah and Nolan worked at different hospitals, so they never crossed paths while working. They agreed that was probably just as well; they both knew of physician/ nurse relationships that were disastrous,

"I could tell you of a number of nurse-physician relationships that began romantically but degenerated into almost civil war. When, following a split, such 'couples' have to continue working in the same environment; it's almost unbearable," said Sarah, somewhat wistfully.

Sarah had experienced her own romantic relationships, but in school they were never serious. She found that most of the male students were interested in drinking and sex, usually in that order, so that they could lose whatever inhibitions and anxiety they harbored. Also, they fumbled around a lot and were very unsure of themselves. She later realized that most of the braggadocio exhibited by young men was a cover-up for their insecurities regarding sex.

One short-term relationship seemed to be heading in the right direction—until she found her guy fooling around with one of her roommates. After giving him the boot, she gave up romance, even dating, for quite a while.

"All of my friends, most of whom were fellow nurses at the hospital, had romantic relationships. They were full of stories, some quite ribald and graphic. Sometimes, I wondered if there was something wrong with me because I didn't have a boyfriend. I could go for months without dating, much less having sex. After a while, I stopped worrying about it. I was so busy with work, and I was a long time in recovery from my last relationship."

Sarah, later on when alone, reflected, *I do find Nolan interesting and physically appealing. He obviously is very intelligent and motivated—characteristics Papa would appreciate. His sense of humor is a little lacking, and he's somewhat surprisingly shy. He's been careful not to force himself on me too quickly. That's unusual for most of the men I have known over the years, who were anything but shy. Most of them just wanted to get laid.*

Nolan and Sarah continued dating, and it became somewhat more serious after several months. Both found the other to be a good conversationalist, and they shared mutual interests. Boating on Lake Pontchartrain was particularly exciting when the wind picked up, and they weren't sure they would make it back to shore safely. They also enjoyed going to college football games. Nolan became an LSU Tigers fan, and Sarah rooted for the Tulane Green Wave. Nolan loved needling her: "How fortunate for your team that it doesn't have to play the Tigers."

Eventually, a more physical relationship developed, mostly by happenstance. Sarah had enough experience to be comfortable with it and eagerly welcomed Nolan's somewhat delayed advances. They found they could enjoy each other sexually without being consumed by it; this made it easier on both of them and was a welcome change from some of their prior romances. They would stay at each other's apartment from time to time, and when their schedules permitted, they would spend several days living together. Neither Sarah nor Nolan was a particularly good cook, so there were a lot of takeout meals. Following a week of going to fast-food diners and bringing pizza or Chinese food back to an apartment, Sarah mused, *If my eventual marriage or at least my living with a man depends on my abilities in the kitchen, there might be a long delay in the process.*

One memorable night, Sarah invited Nolan to spend a weekend in Shreveport at her family home. Sarah felt that advance preparation was a necessity; she needed to explain her family to Nolan, and she was quite concerned about how her parents, particularly her father, would view him. Bringing a West Coast, somewhat socially liberal man to her home was a first for her. She was certain that, eventually, there would be a political discussion between Nolan and her father. Sarah decided to invite her physician uncle, with whom she had a very good relationship, for the same weekend—he could serve as a buffer.

It turned out that her fears were unfounded. James and Nolan bonded almost immediately. It was as if Nolan was the son James had never had—not that he let on to that, particularly around his daughters or his wife. James told his wife,

"You know, for a Northern boy, that Nolan is all right. I think he will do well by our daughter."

James spent most of the weekend showing Nolan around the property, sharing his knowledge of Southern flora and fauna, and "just having a good ol' time." Once Nolan was able to understand James's dialect, with its dramatic Southern drawl—Nolan later joked with Sarah, "Why and how did Southern folks stop using consonants?"—they talked with each other like longtime friends. Sarah eventually had to pry Nolan away from Papa to spend time with her.

"I was wrong! Papa loves you, and so do I!"

After that weekend, it was obvious to each of them that they were likely to spend much more time, possible their lives, together.

CHAPTER 4
Thoracic Surgery

NOLAN GOT THE CALL FROM THE EMERGENCY DEPARTMENT AT 2:00 a.m. A middle-aged man had been brought in by the paramedics with severe chest pain radiating to his neck and back. He was nearly in shock, with a blood pressure of about 60 systolic (the upper of the two numbers of a blood pressure reading). He also suffered from profound weakness on the left side of his body, raising the possibility of an acute stroke. The medics' diagnosis was a heart attack, but when the ER nurses took blood pressure readings in each arm, the numbers differed from each other significantly. An alert ER physician raised the possibility that the patient was suffering from an aortic dissection—a tear in the inner lining of the artery—a severe situation that's often fatal. The tear sometimes blocks blood flow to other arteries, such as those going to the brain (causing stroke-like signs), arms, abdomen, and legs, which could explain the differing arm blood pressure readings.

They took quick blood draws for heart enzymes to evaluate for a heart attack and then did a complete blood count and a portable chest X-ray, which showed a mildly enlarged heart and a little fluid in the chest cavity but nothing else of significance.

When Nolan arrived in the ER, he made a quick assessment and concurred with the ER doctor about the possibility of a dissection. He also heard a loud heart murmur, one like he had never heard before. It was very audible through his stethoscope, occurring in the diastolic, or "resting" phase, of the heart's normal contractions. This signified to him that there was a leak of the aortic valve that was allowing blood to flow backward into the heart chamber, creating the abnormal noise, or heart murmur. That situation, when created by a dissection, had put sudden immense stress on the heart.

After calling a radiologist in to perform an emergency aortic angiogram to establish the diagnosis, he had the nursing staff notify the operating room of potential emergency surgery. Nolan then had every available physician and nurse listen to the poor patient's chest, telling each of them, "You will probably never again hear a heart murmur like this one!" Fortunately, the patient didn't grasp the significance of his statement.

The angiogram confirmed the diagnosis of an aortic dissection, a so-called type I, which extended the tear forward in the direction of blood flow, beginning at the aortic valve. The only reasonable treatment was surgical repair, which itself was a complex and risky procedure. It required placing the patient on cardiac bypass (substituting a machine for the heart during the operation). Only a few major hospitals were equipped with both the manpower training and experience necessary to perform such a surgery. Charity Hospital was one of them.

At the time of this event, spring 1990, Nolan was a senior surgical resident, already on track to becoming a thoracic surgical specialist. In fact, he was to begin his fellowship year in June, at which time he would be in charge of all the residents rotating through thoracic surgery and teaming with senior staff members on all the major cases. He had scrubbed in (the medical slang for operating room activity) on many emergency cases, but this was his first time for a dissection, and he was both excited and apprehensive. Fortunately, the chief of thoracic surgery and the thoracic surgery fellow were both available. By the time the patient was prepared for surgery, the entire surgical team was in place.

When the patient's chest was first opened, one could hear a pin drop in the operating room. Thankfully, the aortic tear had not extended completely through the wall of the blood vessel; that is, it was contained within the aorta. (When the tear extends completely through the wall, the patient usually bleeds to death in a matter of a few minutes.)

"One more hour's delay, and this fellow would have been a goner," said the chief surgeon.

Thirteen hours later, the operation was finished. The patient's aortic valve and a short portion of his aorta had been replaced. The dissection, which extended into the right carotid artery, causing the stroke-like signs, was repaired as well. Blood flow had been restored to all the major vessels, and, thankfully, the blood vessel tear had not extended into the abdomen. The patient was successfully taken off cardiac bypass, his heart restarted, and the surgical incision closed. The patient then was taken directly to the surgical ICU. The exhausted but exhilarated surgical team, including Nolan, accompanied him.

It was a combination of physical and mental exhaustion, mixed with exhilaration. We knew that we had performed well but also that the patient's life remained in grave danger. No one was celebrating, only praying, Nolan later reflected.

For the next ten days, at least one surgical resident stayed constantly with the recovering patient in the ICU. There were a few setbacks, but overall, he continued to recover. Nolan attributed the seemingly good outcome as much to the patient's prior good medical condition (he had mild hypertension for years but otherwise no risk factors) as to the skill of the physicians and nurses. Regardless, this episode was another in a long line of contributing factors to Nolan's maturation as a physician and, in particular, as a surgeon. He was gaining the confidence he knew was required to be as successful in his field as he expected to be.

There was little time for celebration. Surgery at a busy medical center, whether in New Orleans, New York, Chicago, Los Angeles, or anywhere in the world, is a continuum; critically ill patients come and go. Some survive, and others do not. The attending staff rarely draws a satisfying deep breath after a job well done, because there is always another challenge waiting in the wings.

CHAPTER 5
Nolan and Sarah

ANOTHER FORM OF CELEBRATION WAS IN ORDER IN JUNE OF that same year—Sarah and Nolan announced their engagement. Over the course of six years, busy though they were with Nolan pursuing his surgical training and Sarah continuing in her nursing career, they managed to find time together. They had traveled to California so that Sarah could meet Nolan's family, and they continued to visit Sarah's family in Shreveport. Nolan strengthened his relationship with the sometimes overbearing but nonetheless attentive James, who was elated over the engagement. Two of Sarah's sisters were already married and had moved away from Louisiana. James and her mother, Anne, were not-so-secretly hoping that Nolan and Sarah would remain close by.

There was the matter of a wedding. Sarah didn't want a blowout affair but knew that her parents would push hard for one. One of her sisters had followed her parents' wishes with a large celebration on the spacious grounds of the family home; the other had eloped— her parents never understood that decision.

Sarah told Nolan, "Repeating anything in that fashion would kill my parents." So she resigned herself to a big wedding celebration.

There also was the matter of the relationship between Sarah and her mother, Anne. Anne was a throwback to another era, in which a wife was expected to tend the home and raise the children. Anne had never completed her college education; instead, she'd spent all her years as a homemaker. She never complained and seemingly was satisfied with that decision. But her daughters—Sarah in particular—sometimes showed the resentment that came with viewing their mother as subservient to her husband. When the girls raised that specter to their mother, it was often met with a defensive outcry or with a tearful retreat to her personal quarters.

"Sarah, I have never wanted to be anything other than a wife and a mother. It's how I was raised, and I've never seen any reason to change. I don't understand why women nowadays are so dissatisfied with that. I never bought into the sixties revolution, sexual or otherwise. Why do all my daughters fail to understand that?"

"Mother, it isn't that we don't understand you and your attitudes about a woman's role in the world. It's just that you don't understand—don't *want*—to understand *us.* You don't want to see your daughters find a career they believe in. You think that doing so will prevent them from finding a husband and raising a family. Nothing could be further from the truth."

Most of Sarah's friends and other family members were convinced that Sarah was determined to find a career and make her own mark in the world in order to prove to her mother that a woman was capable of doing so.

The wedding took place that summer. And, as expected, it was a lavish and beautiful affair. With magnolias, asters, petunias, and lilacs in bloom and with the sweet scent of honeysuckle in the air and the flavor of mint juleps, how could it be otherwise? Nolan's family—parents; brother and sister; and a few uncles, aunts, and cousins—as well as friends from as far back as high school days traveled a great distance to attend the wedding. Most of Sarah's family and friends were local, so they had it easier. Some of Nolan's and Sarah's medical colleagues, including a few of their instructor from their training days, came as well. Everyone seemed to enjoy themselves, and most said that it was one of the most beautiful events they'd ever been part of. Expectations for the newlyweds were high.

The honeymoon was subject to work-related time constraints, but Sarah and Nolan were able to take five days and drive to Myrtle Beach, South Carolina, which was a Southern-style city in every way. Magnificent trees lined the wide streets, homes had front porches and verandas, and flower gardens had meandering pathways that seemed to continue on forever. Nolan had reserved a suite close to the beach, remote from most of the tourist spots. It turned out to be a good decision, as both Sarah and Nolan enjoyed not only being with each other as a newly married couple but also the peace and serenity of the region.

Sarah said, "I feel like I've just found a spot three blocks from where I grew up." She felt close to her Southern roots and comfortable in that environment. Whether she desired to remain in a similar environment in the future was a decision for another day.

On returning to New Orleans, they again immersed themselves at work. Sarah's hours were somewhat stable and predictable, and she had gained enough seniority within the system to, generally, design her work schedule as she saw fit. For Nolan, however, that was not the case. Surgical training in the United States had always been rigid and relatively inflexible. Designed and implemented by surgical legends like William Halstead and Harvey Cushing, the system was based on intense competition between the residents. The hierarchy, from chief of service down to the lowly first-year resident, was pyramidal—there was room at the top for only a very few of the original cadre of surgical trainees. The competition for senior positions virtually eliminated camaraderie and cordiality; it was often brutal.

Nolan found that, even as a surgical fellow in the last year of training, he remained subject to that rigidity. His hours were long. The only significant benefit was that, when he was on call for emergencies, there was a buffer of junior residents that evaluated individual patients first, before deciding on the necessity of calling him in to operate. That generally enabled Nolan to obtain five to six hours of uninterrupted sleep, something he'd never had in his earlier years of training.

Nolan told Sarah, "I love being a surgeon. But the training process is even more difficult than I was told it would be by my mentors or had imagined myself. Someday, medicine will learn how to train surgeons without subjecting them to overwhelming stress. But I'll never live to see that happen."

During his fellowship year, Nolan developed and refined his skills in the art and science of thoracic surgery. Many of his patients required surgery for relatively common medical conditions, including, unfortunately, lung cancer. New Orleans, like the South in general, was rife with cigarette smoking. Many of the smokers were indigent, very often black or Creole. In addition, members of these same cultures suffered from other debilitating diseases such as diabetes, hypertension, so-called comorbidity factors that increased the likelihood of complications from major surgical procedures. For these and other reasons, Nolan's patients did not fare as well as did patients from more prosperous regions of the country, such as Boston, Salt Lake City, or New York City. When survival statistics were published in the surgical literature, Charity Hospital, along with notable ones such as Cook County Hospital, Chicago, or Columbia University Hospital in New York's Harlem district, often looked dismal by comparison. Only the medically sophisticated understood the reasons for that.

Nolan developed a friendship with the other thoracic surgery fellow, Philip Rivers. Nolan and Phil spent a lot of time together, not just in the operating room but also off duty at the local watering holes that were pervasive in New Orleans. Sometimes, their conversations revolved around the people they were caring for at Charity.

"Phil, it just blows my mind that so many of our patients are completely blind to the risks they take—heavy cigarette smoking, drinking to excess, not controlling their weight or their diabetes. Why don't they understand what they're doing to their bodies?"

"You don't have a clue," Phil said. "These people are at the very bottom of the socioeconomic pool. They have never been educated as to medical risks. Their role models are just like they are and have been that way for generations. Everyone around them does the same thing; there's no reason for them to change. Until we break the cycle of ignorance, nothing will change."

Unlike Nolan, Phil was a product of an economically disadvantaged urban environment, the very same type of community as the one he was charged with providing medical care for. He knew that Nolan's naive attitude in regard to the disadvantaged people in New Orleans would only slowly evolve. Curiously, that was true in spite of the time that Nolan had spent in San Francisco, a city with its own socioeconomic problems.

In spite of his lack of understanding of inner-city socioeconomic problems, Nolan grew increasingly confident in his surgical skills. He and a few of his mentors felt he lacked the emotional skills to deal with the patient and their families when confronted with serious surgical problems and the decisions to be made. He often found himself unable to explain, in simple English, what the patient could expect from the surgery and what the long-term outcome might be. Nolan recognized these personal deficits and took pains to correct them and to enlist help from others. That included his wife, Sarah.

"Sarah, you are so much more skilled in relating to people than am I. I would love it if you could teach me how to be more effective. Would you consider involving yourself with some of my patients and their families? I'll follow your lead and example; maybe it will help me to become a better physician."

"I'd be happy to try, Nolan. I don't know for sure that I'll make that much of a difference to you in the long run, but I'll certainly make the effort."3

He obtained permission for her to accompany him to Charity to meet with patients and their families and to learn what they knew of their current medical situations. Then maybe she would be able to explain whatever they might not have understood.

Sarah proved to be very effective. Other surgeons took note of this somewhat novel approach and began requesting similar assistance from social workers or the nursing staff—anyone who might be willing and able to help them to relate to the patients and families.

Nolan was certainly grateful and expressed his gratitude to Sarah many times over the course of several years. He also said to her, "When I have the time, I'm going to write to UCSF's medical school and suggest that they include at least one course in 'doctor and patient relationships' in their curriculum.

There is no indication, however, that Nolan did so. He was just too busy trying to learn how to become a competent surgeon.

CHAPTER 6
Transition

DURING HIS FINAL YEAR AT CHARITY HOSPITAL, NOLAN BEGAN the process of deciding where to establish his surgical practice. The amount of time and work necessary to arrive at the right decision was significant and particularly stressful, as he had to do it while continuing his duties as a thoracic surgical fellow. He also now needed to discuss it with Sarah and include her in the decisionmaking process. Where would she like to live? Did she wish to continue her nursing career? (He expected that she would.) And importantly, what type of practice was he going to consider? Private practice, academic, a combination of both?

"Nolan, the most important thing for me is that you are satisfied with your decision," Sarah told him. "You've put a lot more time and effort into preparation for your career than I have. You'll have to spend whatever time and effort is necessary to make the right decision, and I'll back you, whatever you decide."

"Sarah, you know me well by now. You know that I need your assistance. I don't want to make that decision by myself. Promise me that you'll help me and that we'll do it together."

Sarah told him that she would become involved in the decision.

In his earlier days, Nolan was certain he would pursue an academic direction, but that had changed over the years. He loved the surgical arena and realized that academics involved a host of administrative duties, which would detract from his time in the operating room. Also, Nolan had learned how stressful it was for academicians to advance in the university hierarchy, which required one to perform research and publish papers with regularity—the "publish or perish" phenomenon. Those were not his major interests or his strengths. And there was the question of finances—he knew that he would make substantially more money in private surgical practice. Nolan knew of many surgeons who earned $500,000 or more a year, a substantial sum at the time. It wasn't that he had expected to become wealthy as a physician; he had always felt that medicine was more about taking care of people, the self-satisfaction that came with it, and obtaining the public's high regard. On the other hand, Nolan was becoming a little more realistic (or sanguine), knowing that having a high income would allow him many opportunities he might not enjoy if he pursued an academic career.

"I want to be able to provide for you and—hopefully, one day—our family. You grew up with all the advantages of a high economic status, and I don't want you to have to give that up."

"Nolan, don't lay that on me. If making a lot of money is important to you, then come out with it. I don't need coddling. I don't need all the material things that my parents have. If you believe that you do, then be honest with yourself and with me."

Nolan listened carefully to Sarah; he was somewhat surprised, however, by her vehemence—the way she threw the "money thing" back into his lap. He didn't bring it up for discussion again.

Nolan began the private practice interview process. Sarah, who had spent her entire life in the South, was nevertheless willing and even eager to try something different. That could include living in other regions of the country, but she hoped to stay, as she told him, "east of the Rockies," so as to be within a relatively short plane trip to visit her family. Nolan would have liked to have included the San Francisco Bay area but decided that it was very important that Sarah be happy. She likely would find San Francisco too far from her family and too liberal for her liking.

Nolan also decided that, if he could find a private practice that would allow him to be an attending physician at a nearby university hospital, allowing him to teach part-time, that would be a good compromise. Because he had performed well at Charity and, thus, expected to receive very good recommendations from his professors and attending staff, Nolan searched out high-level medical practices in several urban areas, including Chicago, Saint Louis, Boston, and even New York (though he had difficulty imagining Sarah and him living happily in New York City).

Several interviews followed the usual chain of letters, phone calls, and recommendations. One in particular caught their fancy, a tenperson surgical practice on the outskirts of Chicago on the North Side, which was in the proximity of several high-level universities. Also, the Lakeshore area of Chicago, which they had visited several times previously, was enticing, in spite of the notorious Chicago winters. He met most of the group's physicians over the course of several visits. The travel fare depleted his meager savings, but he considered it a worthwhile investment.

The surgeons were well trained and had good reputations in the area and at two nearby hospitals. Importantly, they had been in an established practice for over twenty years. As well, they promised Nolan that, if everything went as planned, he would be made a full partner within four years. Finally, they would allow him to serve as an active attending university hospital physician for one day every other week, without incurring any financial loss.

Sarah went to Chicago on one of Nolan's visits and immediately found an available nursing position, pending Nolan's acceptance of his own. Nurses with Sarah's experience were highly sought by most hospitals. Sarah thought that she'd had enough of the high-intensity pressure of the ICU and now would become a general ward nurse on a medical service. She became quite excited about the transition, to the point of almost begging Nolan to accept. She also looked around Chicago for housing. She found a beautiful two-bedroom apartment on Lake Shore Drive, with a partial view of Lake Michigan from the balcony. It was more costly than they had anticipated. But, they rationalized, they both would make a very good initial salary, so they could make it (that is, if they could talk James into loaning them the first and last months' rent). "Don't worry, Nolan. I'll be able to handle my father."

Three months later, in June 1991, they left New Orleans, stopped on the way north to say goodbye to Sarah's family, and began the journey to Chicago.

CHAPTER 7
Chicago

THE WINDY CITY HAD ALWAYS BEEN, LIKE ITS BIGGER BROTHER New York City, a melting pot for people from many regions of the country and all over the world.

Originally, Chicago was populated by hunters and traders that took advantage of its location on Lake Michigan, which provided access to the other Great Lakes and its immense forests and population of game animals. It later morphed into a hub for meat processing and shipping. The famous Chicago stockyards, which served as a backdrop for Upton Sinclair's seminal muckraking work, The Jungle, survived for decades. The stockyards served as a place of employment to the hordes of Polish, Slavic, and Italian immigrants who arrived in the mid-nineteenth century, setting up shops and homes that would remain cultural enclaves for decades.

Hundreds of thousands of black Americans arrived from the South following the Civil War and the Reconstruction Era (a misnomer, as the result, in part, of the efforts of President Andrew Johnson, Lincoln's successor, was hardly a "reconstruction" but, rather, a furthering of racism in the still-segregated South). Multitudes of warravished black families migrated to the North in search of work and freedom. Many of them found the former. But somewhat ironically, Chicago ended up as segregated as was the South. Blacks were prohibited (de facto and de jure) from residing anywhere close to the central city, the financial district, or the affluent lakefront region. They ended up congregating in the southern area of the city. These areas became the ghettos of South Chicago and, at the least, de facto segregation that continues to the present day.

Even into the mid-twentieth century and with the coming of the civil rights era, segregation flourished in the North. Ironically, during the 1960s, at the height of the anti-Vietnam War demonstrations and the infamous Democratic Convention riots in Chicago, it was Mayor Richard Daley, Chicago's unabashed oligarch, serving as mayor for twenty-one years, who was responsible for increasing racial tensions. Daley was a Democrat, chairman of the Cook County Democratic Party for twenty-three years but not in the mold of progressives of the time, such as Eugene McCarthy, George McGovern, or Robert Kennedy. Rather, Daley was more interested in maintaining the status quo for Chicago, and that included racial division.

None of this was of concern to Nolan or Sarah when they arrived in Chicago. Like virtually all people who moved to a chosen region, they were concerned only with a good beginning. Excited about the location of their beautiful apartment and eager to begin their medical careers, they were oblivious to any of the sociopolitical background. They did find time, however, to explore the city. They cruised Michigan Avenue, with its fashionable stores and upscale restaurants on a sunny day, enjoying the varied cuisine. In particular, they enjoyed the nightlife, like listening to Chicago jazz on legendary Wabash Avenue and State Street. Chicago legends such as Buddy Guy and Cannonball Adderley took the music of Southern greats Louis Armstrong, Ella Fitzgerald, Fats Waller, and Count Basie and developed their own styles, and were soon recognized as among the greatest of American musicians. Sarah, in particular, was an avid jazz fan, with her Southern roots and knowledge of its musical heritage. She was skeptical at first but soon grew to love the musical sound that had become the "Chicago Blues" to the world.

Sarah told Nolan, "I grew up in the South listening to white-boy music. My first musical icons were Elvis, Buddy Holly, and Pat Boone. If I ever heard music by Ray Charles, Ella, or Chuck Berry, it was accidental, since most deejays in the South shunned their music. It just wasn't the sound that most Southern kids wanted to hear or, importantly, that their parents wanted them to hear."

Chicago culture also thrived in the museums, such as the Chicago Art Institute and the Field Museum. But Sarah was partial to live theater, and when she scored orchestral section tickets to *Les Misérables,* she was ecstatic. As a literature major in college and an avid reader all her life, she had read Victor Hugo's novel. She never, not in her wildest dreams, thought that such a spectacle, with its post-French Revolution battle scenes and human carnage, could be staged so dramatically and spectacularly. She returned to the theater three times, dragging Nolan twice, and when he finally begged off, she took one of her nursing buddies. Her immersion into Chicago lifestyle was total.

It was not difficult for Nolan, in the meantime, to immerse himself into his surgical practice. His physician associates and the staff in the office were accomplished, and they took pains to make him feel welcome and part of the team. At the two hospitals at which he attended, it was similar—excellent facilities with top-notch nursing care, ancillary support personnel, and very well-equipped, state-ofthe- art operating theaters. Modern structures, they were a far cry, aesthetically, from the aged buildings of Charity Hospital.

After a short time in medical practice, Nolan reflected on his experience so far. *I was blown away by the facilities in Chicago's hospitals. It was like taking a voyage into the future—air-conditioned operating rooms with purified aeration to limit infections; glistening tables; bright walls that replaced the drab gray walls of old-style hospital rooms; and nurses and doctors wearing multicolored caps and masks, making them look like actors in Shakespeare's* Midsummer Night's Dream. *They were capable, well-trained caregivers, who performed as well as any of the academically aligned providers with whom I had trained. It was a real awakening for me.*

It took some time for Nolan to develop the referral pattern from the general practitioners and internists that was necessary to direct patients to him. That was the normal pattern for young physicians who were getting established in a community. During the initial months of practice, he mainly functioned as an assistant for his colleagues. That wasn't a problem, as all of them were accomplished surgeons in their own right. He even added to his own bed of knowledge while assisting on a number of complex cases.

Eventually, over the course of a couple of years, he established his own practice. By the time he was made a full partner, he had gained the trust and confidence of many community physicians. Some of them began referring directly to him instead of several of his colleagues. That could have been problematic, but Nolan took great pains to maintain his partners' trust. He never accepted patients who had previously been cared for by one of his partners, as he believed that was highly unethical.

He told Sarah on one evening, "I had a patient who wanted me to do the follow-up surgical procedure to a pneumonectomy (lung removal). This guy didn't care for one of my partners who had performed the surgery, even though the outcome was fine. I had to refuse him; all I need is for my partners to find out that I was 'stealing' their patients!"

At the university hospital where he became an adjunct clinical instructor in thoracic surgery (academic wording that usually denoted an unpaid position), Nolan quickly learned to differentiate the level of competency of the young residents, interns, and nurses he supervised in the operating room and on the wards. It was a fine art of instructorship to find the correct blend of supervision and independent decision-making for the residents. Of course, major mistakes, particularly in the operating room, could not be permitted, but decision-making was another matter. Every budding surgeon had to develop his or her own style and confidence to function in the real world of surgery, and Nolan spent an inordinate amount of time and mental energy dealing with that process.

During one particularly difficult surgical case, involving an elderly patient who had undergone a prior thoracotomy (surgical opening of the chest), a senior resident was having difficulty dissecting to access the lung lobe that was to be removed. That was because extensive scarring had developed from the prior surgery. The resident was noticeably shaken. Nolan, performing as the first surgical assistant, allowed the resident to continue the dissection unimpeded. But suddenly, a significant amount of bleeding began inside the chest cavity, enough that the entire surgical team, as well as the attending anesthesiologist, were startled and reacted reflexively in response to the hemorrhage.

By the time Nolan had found and isolated the severed artery that caused the bleeding, the patient had lost at least one unit (500 cc) of blood, and his blood pressured had dropped. The anesthesiologist increased the rate of intravenous fluids and administered plasma to stabilize the patient. The operation resumed to completion, but the patient was taken to the surgical ICU postoperatively, due to his labile status. Following a stormy ten-day course, he recovered.

All surgical complications (and this was one) are automatically reviewed by a committee of surgeons of the involved hospital staff in virtually every hospital in the country. This is known, somewhat gruesomely, as the morbidity and mortality conference. In this particular case, the chief of thoracic surgery chaired the committee. At the meeting, Nolan was called to discuss the complication and his role in it. The chief made his displeasure known, chastising Nolan somewhat severely in front of many attending physicians for what he felt was "lack of responsible supervision of a surgical resident."

Nolan did his best to explain what had happened—how he had watched carefully as the resident operated and that he, Nolan, had dealt with the problem immediately. But the chief was not satisfied and made it clear that Nolan's function as an adjunct professor was in jeopardy, and his status would be reviewed again in three months' time.

Nolan was devastated. For several weeks, he thought of little else, even while operating on his own patients. He discussed it with Sarah, who reassured him that he had acted wisely and professionally.

She suggested that Nolan ask to meet again, one-on-one, with the chief of the service. "You have to present your side directly to your chief. I'm sure that, once he has listened to you in a one-to-one discussion, he will understand what you were trying to do—allowing your protégé to make the right decision, without endangering the patient."

"Sarah, I already presented my side of the case at the committee meeting, but it was to no avail. I'm not going to beg. If they don't agree with me, they have every right to reprimand me. I'll just take my lumps and move on."

Nolan was injured emotionally and was too proud to "beg." He continued on as before but not with the same verve and satisfaction that he had previously experienced as an instructor. It was the first time in his career—in fact, in his life, as far as he could remember—that he had been reprimanded so severely. And to make matters worse, most of his colleagues and those at the university hospital knew about the entire sordid affair. He could see it and could feel it in the air whenever he entered a ward or the operating room. And it hurt.

Teaching in medicine had been one of Nolan's primary goals when he'd decided to go to medical school. Now, this dream was in chaos. Nolan began to question whether he should continue in his position as a clinical instructor.

CHAPTER 8
Sarah, Reflecting

SARAH WASN'T SURE ABOUT ALL HER OWN DECISIONS. HER position as a nurse on the medical floor, though at times rewarding, lacked the immediacy and quick decision-making that she had experienced as an ICU nurse. It was a matter of balance, or unbalance, as the case might be. On the positive, her hours were, for the first time in her career, regular and predictable. She was able to plan her days, to get around the city, and to shop when she felt like it. The fatigue that had often overcome her in her previous role was gone. Sarah realized, after leaving the ICU staff, that many of the nurses she'd left behind were younger than she was. Although only twenty-eight, she felt like the old lady of the group. Being an ICU nurse was definitely a job for the young and energetic.

The negative aspects of her new position were real, however. Many of her responsibilities were relatively mundane—doling out medication, attending to patients' personal hygiene, and making daily entries in the nursing section of the charts. And although she did enjoy being able to converse with patients and their families, even that could become tedious. Trying to answer their medical questions, some of which she felt should have been answered by the patients' physicians rather than her, was often difficult. She found herself being evasive or ambivalent at times. She would sometimes daydream, thinking about her previous life in New Orleans and wondering if she would ever again obtain the same satisfaction that came with truly making a difference in her patients' lives.

Sarah often thought about her decision to scale back on her nursing commitments. *I thought I was burning out, that I couldn't function at the rapid pace I'd been doing for many years. Now that I've changed roles, I'm not sure that was the right decision either.*

Nolan really didn't have anything to do with it, as Sarah readily admitted to herself. She knew he would be supportive whichever way she went in her career. She had a sneaking suspicion that he really didn't care whether she even worked at all, but she didn't go so far as to blame him for her ambivalence. *Whatever decisions I make regarding nursing are mine alone, she told herself.*

And then it happened. Two years after Nolan and Sarah came to Chicago, she was pregnant. It wasn't a great shock—she had given up birth control measures several years ago. When her pregnancy was confirmed, Sarah switched gears and began to plan for her life's next phase. She was excited, and she looked forward eagerly to becoming a mother.

Nolan, more surprised than Sarah, was nonetheless excited as well. He had always known that he would become a father one day but just hadn't spent much time thinking about when that might happen. Now that it was a coming reality, Nolan also realized that his life would change dramatically, though probably not as much as Sarah's would. After all, both Nolan and Sarah were raised in traditional households, where the father continued on with his career, and the mother was primarily responsible for the home front. He didn't see that part changing very much, at least for him.

Many of Sarah's friends, including those who were nurses, were mothers as well, and Sarah envisioned that she could return to work following a pregnancy leave. The hospital where she worked had a three-month leave program and even allowed for a longer, though unpaid, period for new mothers before returning. Sarah, with Nolan's support, would most certainly avail herself of that opportunity.

Sarah's pregnancy went well. She had only minor nausea during her first trimester and no symptoms to speak of after that.

Although she felt, in her own mind, *as big as a house* during the eighth and ninth months, that was typical for any woman at that late stage of pregnancy. The fact that Sarah was only five foot three didn't help that matter. "I envy taller, gangly women who don't even look pregnant in their eighth month!" she said. "Nolan, if I get any bigger, you are going to have to cut a larger entrance in the front door!"

"Don't worry about it, honey. I've got a good power saw and could do it in a minute. Just kidding, of course. You look great. And pretty soon, you'll be back to your normal trim self."

"Right," she said, somewhat mournfully.

She continued to work into the beginning of the ninth month and then took a few weeks off to prepare. She loved and had complete faith in her obstetrician, a woman who actually had trained at Charity Hospital, so there was a special bond between them.

Sarah's delivery of a six-pound, four-ounce boy was uncomplicated. Although Sarah had undergone several ultrasound exams during her pregnancy, she was decidedly old-school regarding knowing the baby's sex in advance. She and Nolan chose to be surprised, knowing that they would be elated either way. They named him James Henry, after both grandfathers, settling the matter of which name would be first by a coin flip. Sarah's father won out.

Since their current apartment had two bedrooms, there was no problem remaining where they were living. The second bedroom was turned into a nursery, resulting in Nolan's study being relegated to an alcove adjacent to the living room. No problem for Nolan, who usually did his reading and case preparation work at his easy chair in the living room anyhow.

For the first three months, Sarah stayed home. She had help from each grandmother, as well as from a visiting nurse. When she eventually decided to return to work, they hired a nanny for daytime care. Sarah's schedule allowed her to be home every night.

And so it went for the next two years. Nolan advanced to partnership and was, thus, secure financially. He had a reliable group of referring physicians and had no problem obtaining enough referrals to keep him busy. He also worked his way onto several medical staff committees, thereby assuring that he would have a say in many of the hospital decisions that would affect his practice.

Although he continued on as an adjunct professor of surgery at the university, he hadn't regained his confidence or satisfaction with it because of the previously discussed "incident."

Only on occasion would Nolan allow himself to ponder whether he was truly satisfied with the direction his medical career had taken. *I never planned to make this much money. I had hoped I would provide care to at least some less fortunate people. I guess that I didn't weigh all the options, such as staying in San Francisco on the staff at the General.*

When he voiced that sentiment to Sarah, she didn't pick up on his ennui, and that both surprised and bothered him. I probably expect too much from Sarah, he thought. *And I've never really gone out of my way to solicit her advice anyhow, so who's to blame?*

Now, each of them had thoughts and regrets that they dealt with separately, rather than as a couple. They didn't realize, during those hectic years of medical practice and child-raising, how much that might come back to haunt them.

CHAPTER 9
Chicago 2

THE LAKE SHORE DRIVE APARTMENT WAS WITHIN WALKING distance of several of Chicago's most notable cultural and architectural icons—Grant Park, Michigan Avenue, and the Chicago Riverwalk. The latter included views of its famous buildings such as the Wrigley and the Tribune Tower. Nolan, Sarah, and young James spent many a spring; fall; and, when the weather was not too scorching, summer afternoon enjoying their city.

Only since the 1980s had these areas of the city become attractive to both Chicagoans and visitors. Mayor Richard Daley's Chicago Beautification Program made them so. The Chicago River of the nineteenth and first half of the twentieth centuries was polluted to the point that people were warned to not consume fish harvested from it due to dangerous levels of toxins, such as mercury and sulfates. The river itself contained raw sewage that was both a visual and olfactory travesty, which was unresolved until the river drainage was redesigned. That produced a reversal of flow from Lake Michigan into the river. Discharge from industrial plants, including the stockyards and the Chicago Transit System was stopped, and the train yards were rerouted away from Michigan Avenue and the adjacent parklands. Now, one could walk the length of Michigan Avenue (approximately five miles) without seeing or hearing a train or smelling the river!

By the early 1990s, downtown Chicago had become a tourist attraction of worldwide acclaim. The city began to reap the financial rewards associated with the renewal, and its citizens adopted an air of smugness regarding their city, similar to that seen with cosmopolitan cities like London, Paris, and New York City. Nolan, Sarah, and their friends and colleagues became part of the new Chicago scene.

Two of their newly made friends, Greg and Ainsley, were both nursing colleagues of Sarah's. They lived on Ashland Avenue in the west side of the city, about four miles from the city center, or the Loop as it was known. Public transportation had always been relatively good in Chicago, and that permitted Greg and Ainsley to live some distance from the hospital without having to drive to work. Parking in the city was both expensive and often unavailable.

Greg and Ainsley could afford to buy a home in the west side, a fifty-year-old brick structure, nicely cared for but, as was typical in Chicago, situated on a very narrow lot without a yard. They would bring their young son into the city on weekends to play in the park or the beach along Lake Michigan. Often, they would hook up with Nolan and Sarah, and the children fast became good friends, initially babbling and then learning to talk and eventually carrying on more independently, as young children learn to do.

Greg was black, and Ainsley, Caucasian. That mattered not a bit to Nolan or Sarah, although Sarah told Nolan that, initially, she was more aware of the interracial marriage than he was because of her Southern upbringing. There were very few interracial marriages in the South up to that time.

Sarah said to Nolan, "I don't think we can bring Greg and Ainsley back to my home for a visit. My father would not be able to handle it. It would be a remake of the movie *Guess Who's Coming to Dinner?*"

Nolan and Greg hit it off immediately. With similar interests in sports (Greg also had been an accomplished athlete in high school), both became Chicago Cubs fans and enjoyed occasionally going to a Cubs game or just hanging out at one of the local sports bars, nursing a beer, and watching the Cubs or the professional football team, the Chicago Bears, on television. Sarah and Ainsley usually took the opportunity to sneak off with the kids to the local shops or markets.

Sometimes, Greg and Ainsley would invite Sarah and Nolan to their home. This often included a takeout dinner, since everyone was so busy with work or childcare. Mostly, it was a relaxed atmosphere, with both couples interacting in the usual fashion—talking about work, the kids, or Chicago's weather.

It was obvious to all of them that their financial situations were quite disparate. The three nurses made comparable and comfortable salaries, but Nolan's income as a surgeon was in another league. That never came up for direct discussion, but as time went on, Nolan occasionally made a comment to the group, such as, "Isn't this a magnificent view from our lakefront balcony?" or, "I'm thinking about buying a sports car, maybe a Porsche."

When they were alone, Sarah reminded Nolan of the financial differences between the couples and asked him to not say anything about material possessions that might make someone uncomfortable.

After a couple of those reprimands, Nolan would become defensive. "If I can't discuss things that I enjoy with my friends, then what can we talk about?"

"But, honey, don't you see that some of our friends become a little bit quiet when you start talking about material possessions? You never used to do that, and I don't think that you should do it now."

Sometimes an argument ensued. But usually, this was short-lived, and both of them would let it pass without further discussion.

They had other friends. Burt Scott was, like Nolan, a junior member of the surgical partnership. He had joined a year prior to Nolan. And, like Nolan, he had rapidly advanced to full partnership. Burt was the stereotypical surgeon in manners and personality; he was very outgoing and self-assured. Without saying so, he believed that surgeons were godlike and should be placed on a societal pedestal.

In addition, Burt was movie-star handsome. Nolan and others often noticed the admiring looks that seemed to follow Burt as he walked through the hospital, even when he entered the operating room area. The nurses seemed to give him their undivided attention when he was making his patient rounds. Some, Nolan thought, stood a little bit closer to Burt than was probably necessary.

Burt was unmarried but had a girlfriend, Angela. They shared an apartment close to the Burketts on Lake Shore Drive. Since Nolan and Burt were partners of similar age and position in practice, it was only natural that they would begin a friendly relationship outside of the hospital confines. After a time, Nolan invited Burt and Angela to dinner, the first time to a high-end Chicago restaurant and, later, to their home.

Sarah was not taken with either Burt or Angela. She found Burt to be pretentious (though admitted that he was "extremely goodlooking"), and she had difficulty making conversation with either of them. Sarah told Nolan she felt that Burt was condescending to her in particular and to nurses in general.

As for Angela, Sarah told Nolan, "Angela is along for the ride. Being with a handsome surgeon, living on the lakeshore, and being wined and dined at Chicago's finest is a pretty good gig for a girl." Sarah felt that she and Angela had very little in common. Sarah wasn't interested in pursuing a friendship with them. She predicted— correctly, as it turned out—that the relationship between Burt and Angela was doomed to failure.

Nolan quickly realized that a long-lasting friendship between the two couples was not to be, and he slowly began to spend free time with Burt by himself. Sarah was fine with that, though she did make it clear to Nolan where she stood. "Keep your guard up with Burt. He has a roving eye, and I don't want or expect him to get you into trouble."

CHAPTER 10
Financial Opportunity

DURING A RATHER ROUTINE LUNCH IN THE DOCTORS' DINING room, a group of physicians began talking about a plan they were concocting to build a freestanding surgical center. Eventually Nolan became part of the group discussion, and over the course of the next several weeks, he took part in the formulation of the plan.

Freestanding medical centers, owned and operated by physicians and private nonphysician investors, were just beginning to develop throughout the country in the 1980s and 1990s. The primary goal of such centers was obvious to all—the tremendous financial gain that could be derived from them. By removing hospitals from the equation, all the income from the centers' operation would revert to the investors, including the physician partners.

Reimbursement from private insurance as well as public entities— Medicare, Medicaid, veteran organizations, and the like—was divided into two main categories. Part A was primarily composed of hospitals and clinics, laboratories, radiology; and part B consisted mainly of physicians' fees. By far, the greatest amount of money went to part A reimbursement; if physicians and investors could reap some of the reimbursements from part A (such as radiology and lab fees) in addition to the existing surgical fees of part B, the financial gains would be significant.

There were problems with the concept. From the hospitals' standpoint, these centers were in direct competition, and the financial impact on the hospitals would be significant. As well, physicians on the hospitals' medical staffs were guilty, in the minds of the hospitals' boards of directors and administrators, of violating their moral and ethical commitments to provide the best medical care possible without regard to the charges for related services. That was a somewhat specious argument, however, as the hospitals themselves were very interested in financial gain also. Hospitals had been known for driving up costs for pharmacy, radiology, and emergency room departments for years.

Nonetheless, hospitals generally did whatever they could to block or at least impede the development of freestanding centers. The competitive edge that the centers held was significant, primarily related to their lower costs of development and operation, greater efficiency, easier patient access, and less regulatory "interference" than that pertaining to hospitals. Hospitals were reviewed, often annually, by state and federal health care organizations and had to comply with a host of regulations that generally did not apply to freestanding clinics and medical centers.

Nolan and some of his partners, who also took part in the discussions, were ambivalent. Many did not cotton to the idea of competing with the hospitals, which had provided them with everything they needed to practice medicine and perform surgery. The hospitals usually provided nurses, technologists, and other important support personnel, without requiring the doctors to come up with a dime out of pocket. The concept of freestanding, private medical centers was completely new to most doctors and was foreign to everything they knew, both in their training and practice. As well, the physicians would be entering an area in which most had very little, if any, education—the business world. That was intimidating to many of them.

"Times have changed, guys," one of them said. "Reimbursements are decreasing every year. More and more hospitals are buying out physicians, some even making them employees of the hospital. I'll be damned if I spent twelve years in training to have a hospital administrator determine my salary and set my schedule." It was a common sentiment.

"We have to realize the financial risks of setting up and running our own operation," said another. "We'll be in competition with hospitals that have much deeper financial pockets than we ever will have. I'm in favor of the concept, but I'm not too sure I want to be a part of it."

This went on for hours, sometimes over dinner or drinks at a local pub, when the docs opened up after a couple of rounds, and the banter could become testy. But interest in the project remained high.

In spite of reservations, plans for financing and developing the surgical center went forward. In Nolan's own medical group, the split was dramatic, almost down the middle between *for* and *against.* So as to not break the group apart, lawyers were brought in to devise a plan that would allow for those partners who wished to continue their careers as they were doing and also to participate in the center, and those who did not. The partnership meetings to discuss and implement this plan were numerous, long, and often quite contentious. Finally, however, a settlement was reached; Nolan, after much soul-searching and consternation, and in spite of Sarah's more cautious advice, decided to join the "for" team.

A business and financial team was assembled; bank loans (requiring individual partners to assume personal financial liability, a significant risk) were obtained; architects and builders were interviewed and hired; and the surgical center was on its way.

Sarah said to Nolan, "I just hope you don't live to regret this decision. You've always been idealistic regarding medical care; now you're venturing into the investment side of medicine, which I find a little slimy. But if this is what you want, I'll support your effort." "Sarah, you're right about my interests. But you don't understand that the practice of medicine is changing. Costs of running an office are increasing, and surgical reimbursements are decreasing. If I don't look out for our financial interests, no one else will. I promise that this won't change how I practice medicine, though."

CHAPTER 11
Nolan

THORACIC SURGERY HAD BECOME SOMEWHAT ROUTINE AND mundane for Nolan after several years. It is not unusual for physicians to feel that way; so many people enter a field of endeavor, medical or otherwise, with high expectations, believing they will always remain interested and mentally challenged in their work. But reality is different. No job or career is always interesting and challenging, and ennui set in for most, after a while. Nolan was no exception.

Most of Nolan's surgical cases involved the treatment of lung cancer. In a large city with a significant number of cigarette smokers and with a multitude of airborne toxins from industrial waste, it was not surprising that lung cancer would be ubiquitous. Advances in medicine—including the advent of imaging devices such as computed tomography (CT) and PET / nuclear medicine, along with serological studies that broke down cancers into subgroups—allowed physicians to predict outcomes and target therapy more specifically. This made it possible for doctors to determine which patients might benefit from surgery and which would not. In previous years, surgeons began an operation to remove a cancerous lung, only to discover that it was too advanced and could not be removed in its entirely. The morbid medical phrase open and close described those cases that not only proved to be unsuccessful and unnecessary, but also sometimes resulted in postoperative complications, including death.

Nolan was fortunate in that many of his cancer patients did well. Those who had recurrence of their cancer became patients of the oncologists, who often administered chemotherapy; then, Nolan was no longer directly involved with their care. Even when he heard about his former patients from the oncologists, he rarely responded or spent undue time thinking about them. There was no longer an emotional attachment between him and those former patients.

On the other hand, Nolan was making a very good living. In spite of Nolan's concerns, insurance reimbursement for surgical procedures was still very good, even with Medicare, usually supplemented by private insurance, which most of his financially well-off patients carried. He and Sarah had plenty of extra money, which enabled them to do pretty much whatever they wanted to do. In addition, Sarah had continued to work. She kept her earnings in her own bank account and, thus, was able to manage her own finances without having to go to Nolan for money.

Nolan liked it that way. He once told her, "Mom was always having to justify buying anything extra for the house, even though Dad, as a physician, could afford a little bit more. But he ran a tight ship financially, and Mom definitely resented it. My sibs and I didn't like that Mom always had to worry about spending more of 'Dad's money.'"

Growing up in a middle-class household with a physician father, Nolan had never been concerned about his next meal. He'd had his own bedroom in which to escape from his siblings and his parents. There weren't a lot of excess material things, but he'd always managed to get the new baseball glove, a decent bicycle, or a cool T-shirt with a rock star or ball player on the front. Nolan was the typical young man who was trying to find his place in the world without spending much time dwelling on it. He just expected that good things would happen to him and that, one day, he would not have to think twice about spending money for fun things.

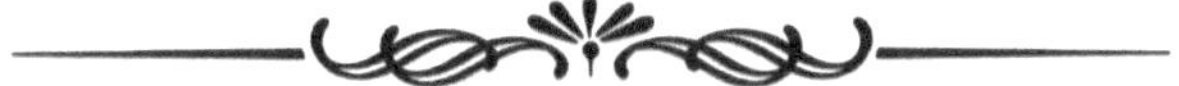

After four years as a clinical instructor, Nolan submitted his resignation to the university. Sarah was puzzled and quite distressed by his action. But when she tried to discuss it with him, he became angry and lashed out at her. "It isn't any of your business!"

"What do you mean it isn't any of my business? My whole life revolves around and depends on us as a couple, on being able to make decisions together. I very much resent your telling me that!"

"Sarah, it's difficult enough as it is trying to balance my practice, start up a surgical center, and teach at the university at the same time. I can't have you or anyone else interfering in how I chose to practice medicine!"

Nolan had never excluded her from a major decision before this. She was severely hurt and distressed by his defiant attitude, and she struggled with both how to manage her anger and how to get through to him, simultaneously.

CHAPTER 12
Nolan and Sarah, Revisited

IN SPITE OF THE ANGST AND OCCASIONAL TURMOIL IN THE Burkett household, both Nolan and Sarah continued with daily duties —their careers, caring for their young son, and looking forward to a more amiable, less contentious marriage.

Sarah's second pregnancy was planned in advance. Sarah and Nolan both wanted for young James to have a sibling for companionship and for learning the art of sharing—always an adventure for a young family. They felt that having two children in a stable home, along with maintaining careers for each of them, would be a good balance. They had ethical concerns as well. Both felt that world overpopulation was a societal concern, and they wanted to address that without hypocrisy. They realized that the days of raising a large family that could help out by working on the farm or in the store or the shop were essentially over. And the previously high infant and child mortality from infectious diseases—typhoid, diphtheria, smallpox—with their resultant reduction of the family workforce was, fortunately, history as well.

Sarah became pregnant again. All went well until the fourth month of pregnancy, when a routine ultrasound exam showed that a placenta previa (the placenta growing over the inside opening of the uterine birth canal) was developing. This condition increases maternal risk significantly, due to the high likelihood of bleeding during vaginal delivery. Therefore, a cesarean section is often necessary.

Nolan was very much in favor of a C-section; Sarah, not so much.

"My natural delivery resulted in a special bonding between me and my baby. I really want for that to happen again."

Sarah, however, reluctantly agreed to accept the C-section if her obstetrician recommended it. And she did.

At the beginning of her eighth month of pregnancy, six weeks before her scheduled C-section, Sarah began to bleed vaginally. She was working at the time, having decided to continue to do so until her ninth month. Fortunately, she was in the hospital where the operation was scheduled, and her obstetrician was available. The Csection was performed without incident that same evening, and the result was a healthy, though somewhat diminutive, baby girl—five pounds six ounces—who would soon be named Jennifer Anne Burkett. In time, that name would be shortened to Jenny.

The Burketts needed more living space now that the family had grown. By 1995, the country had recovered financially from the most recent recession, and real estate property was appreciating significantly. Nolan and Sarah felt it was time to think about buying a home. They had several Chicago areas in mind, all within fifteen to twenty minutes commuting time to work. After seeing a variety of homes, they found one in the Lincoln Park region of Chicago that seemed to answer all their needs—a picturesque area with parks nearby, a well-regarded elementary school, and nearby markets and shops. There was even a police station within several blocks. Sarah liked that, as she had always been concerned about public safety in Chicago.

"I would have liked to have a two-car garage, but I guess that isn't likely around here," Nolan said.

"What do we need with a two-car garage when we have only one car and don't need a second one?" Sarah responded. Sarah was the practical one, and that settled that for the time being.

With Nolan essentially conceding the final decision on home selection to his wife, they bought it and moved in a couple months later. Minor repair work followed, nothing too dramatic—outfitting the nursery and a second bedroom for James, and they were good to go.

Nolan knew he would miss the lakefront view from the apartment but rationalized that they would make the short trip to Lake Shore Drive frequently, and that would have to do.

Nolan kept busy at the hospital and, when not operating, with his office practice. The cases kept on coming, and his overall satisfaction index remained stable, if not tremendous. He also increased his involvement with hospital staff positions, including a stint as medical staff secretary. He believed this was a stepping-stone to being elected chief of the medical staff one day; that was the most prestigious and potentially influential hospital position for a staff physician, and he coveted the position, with its resultant recognition. Recognition and authority became increasingly important and meaningful to Nolan. He wasn't sure why that was, but he accepted the acclaim that would inevitably occur.

Nolan told Sarah one evening, "If I ever become the chief of staff, I'll have a chance to reorganize some of the specialties so that the hospital can reap the benefits that come with recognition for excellence in a given area, such as lung cancer diagnosis and therapy. Right now, we're just performing as individuals; we need to develop a program that will give us recognition."

One day, after a particularly difficult surgery, he was in the ICU with a postoperative patient when a nurse he hadn't seen before approached him with the patient's chart and began to discuss the case. Something about her manner and her way of standing very close to him while speaking seemed somewhat unusual to him. But he let it go, not thinking about it further.

Several days later, a most unusual situation occurred. Nolan was again in the ICU. When he finished making rounds, he needed to use the restroom. He walked to the staff restroom down the hall and opened the unlocked door. As he did so, the same nurse he'd encountered days earlier stood up from the toilet and slowly pulled up her nursing uniform pants.

Shocked and embarrassed at having intruded, Nolan quickly muttered, "I'm sorry," and turned to leave. As he did so, however, he saw the nurse smile in a way that made him think she was not upset in the least by what had happened.

The very next day, when he was again making rounds in the ICU, that same RN gave him a knowing smile and said matter-of-factly, "Don't worry about what happened yesterday. Maybe it will happen again."

Nolan was tongue-tied, but did manage to say, "Well, it certainly doesn't bother me that it happened, since it didn't upset you. In fact, I have replayed the scene visually several times now!"

It took Nolan a long time to put that out of his mind. He even thought about it at night while he was drifting off to sleep, during surgery, and whenever he approached the ICU. This was the first time since his relationship with Sarah had become serious that he had even thought about another woman. Like most men, he had gazed appreciatively at an attractive one in passing, but that was the extent of it. This time was a little different, but he did everything he could to keep any untoward notions or ideas from entering his mind.

Something was bothering Sarah, but she was damned if she could figure out what it was. She was now a mother of two healthy, active children. Her marriage, even with its occasional rocky moments, was at least satisfactory. She had a career, and even though it might not be as exciting as it had been when she'd lived in New Orleans, she realized it had been her choice to reduce the previous level of stress.

There were days when she was depressed. She knew all about the clinical syndrome of postpartum depression; her mother had suffered from it, without really knowing it by name, sometimes retreating into her bedroom for days on end. It had taken a toll on her family, particularly the children. Her father had either ignored or resented her mother's anxieties and was of little assistance to his wife or the family.

Sarah had always taken great pains to separate herself, both physically and emotionally, from her mother. She had decided very early in her life that she would have a career and would be an independent, self-supporting woman, even while raising a family. She would be able to make her own way in the world, if necessary. When she suffered those occasional bouts of withdrawal and melancholy, she made every effort to pull herself out of the doldrums. But she wasn't always successful in doing so.

Sarah didn't feel she needed professional help, but she did rely on her friends, especially her nursing colleagues. At least two of them had gone through similar situations and were eager to provide Sarah with understanding and compassion. One of the women, Zoe, was particularly helpful.

"What you need is some time away from all this," Zoe said. "You need a chance to be by yourself, to think, and to reflect on your life."

"How can I do that," Sarah asked her, "with a husband and two children at home and with a job?"

"You just need to do it. Take a sabbatical from work. Tell your husband you're going away for a week or two and that he'll have to manage. Hire a nanny for the kids and tell Nolan he should consider taking a leave of absence from work while you're gone."

It never worked out that way. When Sarah broached the idea with Nolan, he became defensive and challenged Sarah to explain why she felt as she did.

"I can't explain it fully to you, Nolan. I don't even understand all of it myself. Maybe it's a genetic defect; I don't know. All I do know is that I'm not myself right now, and I feel like I need a little time by myself to get it together."

"I just don't get it, Sarah. You have two wonderful children. You have a career. You have a beautiful home in a terrific neighborhood. What more could you want?"

Sarah thought it interesting and revealing that Nolan had not said, "You also have a loving husband who would do anything to help you."

"For starters, Nolan, I'd like to have a husband who tries to understand that I'm going through a difficult emotional time right now and who makes an attempt to recognize that. I'd like to have a husband who might console and comfort me when I'm down, rather than ignore me and continue on as if nothing is happening to me."

CHAPTER 13
The Storm

A FRANTIC NURSE BURST INTO THE OPERATING ROOM WHERE Nolan's surgical team was finishing an operation. She was very upset but approached Nolan cautiously. In a calm but tearful manner, she said, "Dr. Burkett, you must come out of the OR now and speak with several people who are gathered in the waiting room."

Nolan had never been summoned from an operating room prior to completing a procedure; he knew immediately that something was dreadfully wrong. Pulling off his surgical mask and gloves, he walked hurriedly toward the waiting room, where a group was gathered at the far end of the room. Two were Chicago police officers, another was a hospital administrator who Nolan knew well, and a fourth was the surgical recovery nurse supervisor.

One of the police officers approached Nolan. In a controlled but shaky voice, he said, "Dr. Burkett, there has been an accident involving your wife and family. Your wife and son are mildly injured, but your little daughter died at the scene."

As Nolan tried to comprehend what the officer was saying, he heard the woeful groans from the other people in the group. He found himself gasping for breath, almost collapsing, before the second officer grasped him tightly and sat him down on a nearby sofa.

After a few moments, he gathered his thoughts and began asking questions, most of which he would not be able to recall in the days and weeks that followed.

"Where is my family? Where did the accident happen? When can I see them?"

A police car was waiting and immediately took Nolan to a nearby hospital, where Sarah and James were in the emergency room, being attended to by several nurses, an ER physician, and a hospital chaplain. The chaplain was sitting at Sarah's side, speaking quietly to her when Nolan arrived.

The scene was heartbreaking. Sarah obviously knew that her daughter had not survived the accident. Nolan learned that Sarah had been driving through an intersection on State Street when a car had run a red light and crashed into the passenger side of her car, a dreadful T-bone collision.

Little Jenny, strapped into her infant seat on the front passenger's side, took the brunt of the impact directly. She never had a chance.

Sarah was inconsolable, saying repeatedly, "Why couldn't it have been me? Why did my sweet, beautiful daughter have to be the one to die, rather than me?"

Sarah had a cut on her right arm that was already bandaged and a mild bruise on her neck, where her seat belt had caught her. Otherwise, she appeared to be uninjured. But her mental state was beyond repair.

Nolan, still in shock and disbelief, had the presence of mind to go to James; embrace him and hold him tightly; and, at the same time, as a physician as well as a father, make a rapid assessment of his son's physical health. He saw that, other than a mild bruise on his arm, he seemed to be unhurt. James had been strapped into the back seat and, miraculously, had not been injured.

The following weeks were horrific. The funeral for Jenny was beyond belief. Men and women, some of whom had never known the child, attended the service, and many were overcome with grief. How could something like this happen to an innocent child? It defied understanding and faith. How could God allow a tragedy like this to happen?

The priest who officiated at the funeral did his best. But what could one say? How did anyone comfort a family that had lost a child? Neither Nolan nor Sarah was particularly religious, but both were raised to believe in a supreme being, one who had concern for all earthly living things. That belief made it even harder to understand how such a tragedy could have happened.

Many religions, including Judaism and some Christian sects, teach that God leaves it to humans on earth to conduct their affairs and does not become involved in their personal daily matters. Even for those who believed that, it nevertheless still was difficult, if not impossible, to accept tragic outcomes such as the Burketts experienced.

Similar tragedies, sometimes on a much larger scale—holocausts, earthquakes, plagues, fires, and the like—had happened since the beginning of time. But at this time, an innocent child had needlessly died, due to negligence; it was determined that the driver of the offending automobile was intoxicated and had survived the crash with minimal injuries. He would later be tried and convicted of involuntary manslaughter and serve a lengthy prison term.

Religion does not usually deal with negligence as it does intent; the former is mostly a judicial concern, whereas intent presents moral and ethical dilemmas.

For his part, Nolan refused to even think about the driver who had killed his daughter. *What good will it do? Thinking about him will not bring my Jenny back. I can't stand it.*

Sarah spent hours, days, and weeks in vivid memory of the horrendous event. She spent considerable time forcing herself to think of her Jenny—how they'd laughed and played together and how Jenny would tug on Sarah's hair and say, "Mommy, I want hair like yours!"

Sarah vowed, *I will remember my precious daughter for the rest of my life. Nothing can take away my memories, in spite of the gut-wrenching pain I feel every day.*

Even young James, only six years old, came to understand that he would never see his sister again.

Family and friends did all they could to support and console Nolan and Sarah, but it was of little help. Sarah's parents did everything possible; her mother remained with her in Chicago for several weeks. Eventually, however, it became clear that her daughter needed some solo time to recover, so she went home to Shreveport.

Nolan's parents and siblings also tried their best to assist and provide emotional support. Nolan's father was particularly involved. He and Nolan had had an uneven relationship for many years. His father had always let Nolan go his own way, with little fatherly advice or interference. Nolan wasn't sure that his father was very interested in him as a person. His father seemed to expect that Nolan would make it on his own. Nolan had decided when James was born that he would have a relationship with his son that differed from his with his own father. He looked forward to spending quality time with his son, whether with schoolwork, athletics, or just horsing around. He would spend more time with James than his father had with him. Now, with the death of his daughter, Nolan began to reassess his feelings regarding his father. He spent considerable time reminiscing on the good times they had spent together, and he realized that he had, for whatever reasons, overlooked or forgotten many of them.

Now, at long last, he and his father talked more openly than they had done for a long time. Ironically, it had taken a tragic episode for each of them to realize what they had lost.

Both Nolan and Sarah went back to work. It was a necessity for each of them, particularly for Nolan, who tried to immerse himself in work to dim his mind's constant turmoil over the loss of his daughter. He would never be able to forget her; nor would he want to. But for his own sanity, he had to occupy his mind with other thoughts. As he often told Sarah, otherwise, he might "go crazy with grief."

Sarah had even more difficulty. Initially, she began working two or three shifts per week, alternating with spending full days at home with James. She was worried that he, at such a young age, would be permanently scarred, both by the loss of his sister and by viewing his parents' sadness, which was so apparent, even to his young eyes.

Sarah was depressed. She knew it, and she tried to overcome it by talking about her daughter with her friends, remembering the mother/daughter relationship that just had begun to blossom. She even sought professional help from a psychologist who practiced next door to her hospital, but this was short-lived. Sarah had difficulty discussing such an emotional matter with a stranger, no matter how well-trained and attentive that person might be.

Try as I might, I just can't explain my grief, my loss, to a total stranger, even if that stranger is a trained psychologist. At the end of the day, she went home to her family and lived her life. *I'm left with my sorrow.*

Sarah's greatest difficulty, unfortunately, was in talking with Nolan. Immediately after the incident, they cried a lot. They tried talking about Jenny and all the fun they'd had together—the trips to the zoo, the carnivals, and the park playgrounds. But it was too painful, and each of them retreated into their separate worlds, trying to gain comfort from quiet and solitude. That too had its drawbacks. The isolation led to recurring bouts of depression and despair. Sarah and Nolan both had difficulty accepting the fact that Jenny would never be with them again.

It affected their intimacy as well. In the early years of marriage, they had both enjoyed their sexual relationship. Each was relatively uninhibited regarding sex and experimented with different ways of expressing their sexuality, even to the point where they would joke with each other: "Do you think that this is a little kinky?" or, "I'm sure glad that our parents don't know about any of this."

As often was the case with marriage, after several years, both the rate and the type of sexual activity began to diminish. Then the jokes between them became, "We'll have to do it tonight, for sure!" or, "Do you think that three times a week is a little excessive?"

After the accident, their sexual activity decreased even more dramatically, to the point of almost disappearing. Sarah was caught in the dilemma of knowing how much Nolan enjoyed sex; for her, not so much. The decision to "perform," as she came to think of it, was problematic. Whether consciously or unconsciously, she found reasons and excuses to avoid sex. It was no longer just the mundane joking—"Not tonight. I have a headache"—but, rather, she would actually becoming physically ill when she thought about sex.

At about the same time, Sarah began taking medication, primarily to reduce her level of anxiety. She started with mild sedatives and an occasional glass of wine and later began experimenting with marijuana. Curiously, Sarah had never done any drugs during her college years, having told Nolan, "Good Southern girls don't do drugs!" Now, the situation was different, and she no longer worried what others thought about her actions; she was just going to take care of herself.

Nolan found other ways to relieve stress. Primarily, this revolved around taking one night a week to go out with his buddies, barhopping or going to a jazz club. His alcoholic intake increased, but not to the point where it hindered him.

On one occasion, he found himself at a club with his old friend Burt Scott. They began to reminisce about the old Chicago days, when their lives had seemed less complicated and their interpersonal relationships had been on more solid footing. Nolan and Burt still liked and trusted one another. Over drinks, they shared their problems at work and with women (Burt's marriage was over by then). After several hours, Nolan knew he had reached his selfimposed limit. As a surgeon, he was quite conscious of how alcohol could affect both one's judgment and performance in the operating room. He previously had never drunk the night before he was scheduled to operate.

As he rose to leave, he said to Burt, "I've seen my share of doctors try to operate after having had a few of drinks. It's not pretty. I vowed I would never put my patients in that dangerous position. I'm going home."

CHAPTER 14
Aftermath

DEBBIE SAW HIM AS SOON AS HE ENTERED THE BAR. NOLAN HAD come after work to meet a friend for a drink, as had become increasingly frequent in the days and weeks following the accident.

She was with another young woman at the bar and called out, "Dr. Burkett! It's Debbie, your ICU nurse! Come over and say hello."

Nolan recognized her immediately as the ICU nurse who was part of the "bathroom incident."

When he approached her, Debbie gave him a cordial but not overly familiar hug. Then she introduced him to her friend Olivia. Since Nolan's colleague hadn't as yet arrived, he decided to stay for a few minutes to chat. Debbie immediately expressed her condolences on the loss of his daughter.

"Of course I knew about it right after it happened. The entire hospital staff was in shock over your loss, as am I."

Nolan thanked her for her condolences and then changed the subject. They chatted for a few minutes about nothing of significance; Olivia excused herself to go to the bathroom. At the same time, Nolan's friend came into the bar, and Nolan said goodbye to Debbie.

As he got up, she said, "Wait a minute. I want to give you something." She took out a card from her purse; it had her professional name and a phone number. "If you ever need to talk with someone about what happened or anything else, please give me a call. I'm a very good listener."

Nolan looked into her eyes for a few seconds and then said, "Thank you. I very much appreciate that offer." And he left to join his friend.

Nolan's mind was in disarray. He knew his marriage was in jeopardy. He had lost his daughter, and his professional life, though reasonably stable, was not exactly what he had expected it to be. Should he further endanger his relationship with Sarah by meeting up with Debbie? He tried to convince himself it was an innocent enough thing to do; after all, Debbie had just offered to listen. What would be the harm in that? He could use someone to listen to him, especially given that he and Sarah were not communicating all that well.

The week following the meeting in the bar, Nolan called Debbie. She was very receptive and invited him to come over to her apartment for a drink and a chat. Nolan accepted.

When Nolan arrived at Debbie's place with a bottle of chardonnay, she greeted him in the same warm but cautious manner. Following a brief tour of the apartment, which was tastefully decorated in a decidedly feminine fashion, they went into the living room. The apartment was small but had a knockout view of Lake Michigan from that room, similar to what Nolan had had in his old apartment. He had momentary pangs of remembrance and smiled when he looked out from the balcony; then he went to sit on the couch.

Over the course of the next ninety minutes, they talked; rather, Nolan talked, with Debbie maintaining a fixed gaze on him and occasionally following up with an appropriate comment. Nolan was impressed, so much so that he opened up about his innermost thoughts in a way he hadn't done with anyone, including Sarah, for years.

"Debbie, nothing in my life has affected me as much as the loss of my daughter. I can't stop thinking about her, about the wonderful times we had together. She is"—he caught himself momentarily stifling a sob—"was the most beautiful, most precious child I have ever known. I still cannot believe she's gone."

"Nolan, there is absolutely nothing I can say that will resolve your grief, so I won't even try. The most that I can do is to listen to you and offer you whatever comforting words I can."

Debbie was anything but the seductress. She was very modestly dressed in a pantsuit and blouse buttoned up to her neckline. Nolan congratulated himself on his correct assessment of the purpose of the meeting.

When they seemingly had exhausted their conversation and had almost finished the bottle of wine, Nolan said, "Thank you for inviting me over, and thank you so much for listening to me so patiently. I'm sorry if I've bored you. I'm particularly upset with myself for not having asked much at all about you, your life, and your career."

"Don't worry, Nolan"—he had asked her to call him by his first name at the first moment. "Don't worry about that at all. I've enjoyed every minute of it, and I hope that I've been some help to you by listening. I also hope that I will see you again soon."

Nolan was confused. Is she giving me a signal that she is interested in me for more than conversation and compassionate reasons?

He briefly assessed the situation and decided that it would be best, for now, to merely acknowledge her comment, which he did. With that, Nolan departed. He remembered her words about seeing him again soon and began to wonder whether he had underestimated Debbie's level of interest in him.

The next meeting at Debbie's, two weeks to the day following the first, was decidedly different. Debbie greeted Nolan with a kiss on the cheek as she put an arm around his shoulder. It was obvious that she had thrown any previous caution to the wind. This time, Debbie was dressed differently, in yellow shorts—not too short but revealing shapely legs that still were tanned in the Chicago autumn. Her halter top was a modest one, as it covered her enough to enable Nolan to look at her without embarrassment.

Debbie opened a bottle of wine, and they began to chat as they had before. After about fifteen minutes, Debbie got up from her chair across from Nolan, came over to him, put her hands on his knees, and separated his legs. She then inserted herself between his legs, pressed up close to him, and said, "Nolan, I'm ready for this relationship to go to the next level. Are you?"

There was little that Nolan could say. He put his arm around her waist, drew her closer, and kissed her, first carefully, and then, when she reciprocated, with more passion. The next thing he knew, Debbie's halter top was off.

When Nolan awoke in Debbie's bedroom several hours later, it was approaching midnight, and he realized that trouble loomed. He hadn't ever returned home at that late an hour for anything other than a surgical emergency. Nolan hurriedly dressed, kissed Debbie on the cheek when she stirred, and left the apartment.

When he arrived home, Sarah was asleep in bed. Whether she had gone to bed early and didn't know what time he got home was never discussed or determined. Something told Nolan that she did know but didn't want to discuss it—and that was fine with him. He quietly undressed; got into bed; and tried, unsuccessfully, to fall asleep.

Nolan continued on with his life, which now had added a new dimension—an affair. He rationalized that he would be able to survive, even prosper, regardless of the complication of carrying on an affair in addition to his career as a surgeon, his involvement with the surgicenter, and his responsibilities as a medical staff officer. There was also the fact that he was a husband

and, not least of all, a father to James, a child who was suffering from the loss of his sister. Nolan did try to spend whatever free time he could manage with James, but it never seemed to be enough. In the back of his mind, he saw himself failing as a father, much as he thought his own father had failed him.

As for his marriage, it suffered in silence. Sarah continued as a mother and a nurse but seemed to have lost the will to work on her diminished relationship with Nolan. Did she know or suspect that Nolan was involved with another woman? It was possible, given her relatively noncommunicative family history, that she did know but did not want to suffer through the trials and tribulations of an encounter with Nolan. Sometimes denial and neglect were easier paths to take, and Sarah seemed to have made that decision.

Sarah told herself, *I just can't deal with yet another crisis right now.*

CHAPTER 15
Cyclone

EIGHTEEN MONTHS LATER, THE GREATER CHICAGO Surgicenter was completed and became operational. It was immediately successful; the community physicians began referring directly to the center, as its physician owners had hoped. In part, this was because of the competitive edge the center held over the nearby hospitals—ready access; outpatient rather than inpatient surgery; and personnel who had responsibilities only for the center, rather than the hospital and its inevitable bureaucracy. The patients appreciated the ease with which their needs were managed.

Gradually, many of the surgeons began performing some of their operations at the surgicenter. Even some of the complex thoracic surgical cases could be managed on an outpatient basis, as there was twenty-four-hour patient observation available. Most everyone in the medical community was extremely pleased—except for the hospitals board of directors and their administrators. The threat, primarily financial, was real and endangered the very existence of their hospitals. They realized that, if they did not take action against the center soon, the hospitals might not survive.

Less than six months after the center was opened, two nearby hospitals (one just across the street from the center) filed a lawsuit against the center and the physician investors who operated it. The suit was complex, but the primary allegation was that the center was providing illegal financial incentives to its patients, some allegedly in violation of Medicare, Medicaid, and some private insurance plans. The hospitals demanded $50 million in compensation. In addition, they indicated that the hospitals would dismiss any physician owner of the center from their hospital staff, mostly for unspecified violations of their responsibilities.

One of those violations was specified, however, and stated that the physicians were not available for emergency care when on call because they were working at the center when needed at the hospital, in violation of the hospitals' bylaws. Whether or not the hospitals possessed the legal authority to remove the physicians from the medical staff would be decided in a court of law.

James was now seven years old and immersed in activities befitting his age—attending second grade in school, playing on a soccer team, and spending time with his friends in the neighborhood. Sarah devoted as much time as possible to him, including volunteering as a den mother for his Cub Scouts. She put pressure on Nolan, subtle initially but stronger eventually, telling him, "Our son needs you to be involved at this developmental stage of his life. Can't you try to find a little more time for him?"

"I'm trying to, but my responsibilities at work are overwhelming right now. Once this lawsuit has concluded, I promise I will become more attentive to James's needs."

"You seem to have forgotten what you used to tell me often—that your father was not there for you in your early years, when you really needed him. I just don't understand why you don't heed the promises you made back then, regarding spending time with your children."

Nolan had nothing to say about that. He knew that he was abrogating parental responsibility and forgetting about what he had promised himself in that regard.

Nolan and Debbie's affair continued. Somehow, Nolan was able to find time for it. Whatever guilt he felt when making excuses to Sarah for not being home during evenings was assuaged by the immense pleasure he obtained from his relationship with Debbie. She made him feel as if he was on top of the world whenever they were together. Their sexual activity was innovative and fulfilling, and he couldn't imagine giving it up. Even though he professed to still be in love with Sarah, he felt himself also loving Debbie. But he knew he would never choose between the two of them. Sarah was his wife, and he would remain with her, if at all possible.

One warm May afternoon, Nolan told Sarah, "Burt and I are staying late this evening for a surgicenter meeting. Don't fix dinner for me or wait up for me."

Early that evening, young James developed a fever and began vomiting profusely. Sarah was used to this sort of thing at work, but when it involved her son, an emotional component was involved. She needed Nolan's help.

Sarah didn't have a way to reach Nolan—cell phone not yet available, and beepers and pagers were only to be used by medical personnel. She decided to call Burt's home; he was now married, but Sarah didn't know his wife, Naomi.

When Naomi answered, Sarah introduced herself and said, "Do you have a way to reach Burt at the meeting?"

After an awkward pause, Naomi responded, "Burt's right here. I don't know about any meeting, but you can speak to him if you'd like."

When Burt got on the phone, he said, somewhat hesitantly, "I don't know anything about a partnership meeting this evening."

Sarah ended the conversation abruptly. Sarah experienced a range of emotions over the next several hours. Initially, there was the shock of discovering that Nolan had lied to her about the meeting. That was followed by the realization that he was covering something up, and the most likely possibility was that there was another woman involved. She alternated between fury, sadness, and confusion.

Sarah was also busy attending to her ill son, making James comfortable and getting him bedded down for the night. Finally, she lay on her own bed, trying to sort out her thoughts. *How am I going to confront Nolan on this? Do I initially pretend I know nothing and ask him how his evening was, allowing him to spin a web? Or do I immediately go at him, telling him I know about this lying and demand an explanation?*

It was difficult; she often went to great extremes to avoid confrontation. That had been the case from the time she was a little girl, trying to maintain emotional distance from her siblings and her parents. But this was different. She had a husband who was possibly unfaithful and a son to raise. What was the right approach?

Sarah didn't come to a decision until Nolan walked into the bedroom at around eleven o'clock. His half smile and, "Hello, dear," turned to a quizzical expression when he saw Sarah lying in bed, teary-eyed. He knew there was a problem as soon as she spoke. "I hope you had an enjoyable evening," she said in a shaking voice. Nolan did not attempt to confabulate. He sat down on the edge of the bed and said, "What do you know? And to whom have you been speaking?"

"It's not your business to know how I found out about you, but I do demand to know what you have been doing tonight. While you're at it, what has been happening on the other nights when you have supposedly been attending surgicenter meetings?"

For the next ten minutes, their conversation included a combination of anger (mostly Sarah's); Nolan's attempted explanations (which fell flat); and remorse, poorly delivered. By the end, Sarah stood up; told Nolan he should leave the room, and suggested he prepare "for the worst," which she did not further define.

Nolan made another attempt to explain himself. But by then, Sarah was convinced that, indeed, there was another woman, and she rebuffed him severely, saying, "I don't plan on staying here. Tomorrow I will leave this house with our son and go to my family in Shreveport."

She was not bluffing. The next morning, she packed a suitcase for herself and James, hailed a taxicab, told James to bid goodbye to his father, and left.

James, still ill, nonetheless knew something bad had happened and cried, "Mommy, Daddy, where am I going? Why isn't Daddy coming with us?"

Nolan did not want his son to see an argument between his mother and his father. He knelt down in front of James. "Don't worry, son. I'll be with you soon. For now, just be a good boy, and do whatever your mother asks of you."

Following three days and nights without more than a moment's sleep, Nolan requested an emergency leave from his medical practice. His partners knew something major had occurred but not what it was. They had watched his behavior and performance for those few days, however, and were alarmed as well as concerned for him. One of his associates who had operated with him the previous day told his partners that Nolan's attention was compromised in the operating room and that he was a risk to his patients. They demanded that he not perform surgery until he could demonstratethat he had resolved whatever was disturbing him. They were relieved when he requested a leave of absence.

Nolan tried, unsuccessfully, to contact Sarah. The first telephone call to her Shreveport home was predictably traumatic. When her father, James, answered the phone, there was a long pause, after which James told Nolan that his daughter did not wish to speak with him and that he, Nolan, should not call back.

Nolan tried to get James to listen to him. "I need to talk with Sarah," he insisted. "I want to come to Shreveport to see her."

James laughed in a harsh, pungent manner. "You are not welcome at our home. You've betrayed my daughter and broken her heart. Given the circumstances, my wife and I will not allow you not set foot in our home again."

Nevertheless, Nolan called back each day for the next week. One time, he was successful in getting his son on the line, and they talked for several minutes. James told his father that, although he was getting along well, he wanted to see him.

Nolan suppressed a cry and told his son, "We will certainly see each other very soon."

"How soon?" James asked.

Nolan could not answer.

Ten days after the catastrophic event, Sarah relented and took Nolan's call. They spoke briefly, during which time Nolan attempted another apology for his behavior and pleaded with Sarah to return home. He needed to talk with her in person, and he wanted desperately to see his son.

Sarah told him that she was willing to return but gave no indication that she was willing to resume their prior relationship.

Their reunion was tense. Following the perfunctory greetings and Nolan and James's tender embrace, Sarah and Nolan had a long private talk on the patio of their home.

Sarah had been thinking about how she wished to handle the situation and had decided she was not interested in hearing the details of Nolan's affair—with whom, how had it begun, whether it was a serial set of events, and so forth. She was interested, however, in hearing from Nolan was how he planned to go forward— whether he was strongly motivated to cease and desist in this and any future affairs and how he could demonstrate to her that he was being truthful.

Nolan was contrite. He too had spent a lot of time thinking about what to say to Sarah and, most importantly, what he was going to do about his relationship with Debbie. He was glad Sarah hadn't demanded details; that would be too difficult for him to discuss. Besides making another feeble apology, the best thing he did was to say he would gladly join her in meeting with a marriage and family counselor. That was the first time he had received any semblance of a positive vibe from her since the beginning of the sordid affair, and they decided they would go forward with counseling.

CHAPTER 16
Debbie

DEBBIE FOUND OUT ALMOST IMMEDIATELY THAT NOLAN'S WIFE had discovered his infidelity. Nolan called her the day after his encounter with Sarah and told her, in a shaky, broken manner, "Sarah knows about us and is completely destroyed and threatening to leave me."

Debbie was not shocked to hear it. She had heard murmurs of gossip among her hospital colleagues. One had said to her, "There's an affair involving one of our nurses and a well-known surgeon." And Debbie expected that it would break out into the greater community before long. Her immediate reaction, following attempts to console Nolan and find out what he planned to do, was to figure that out for herself.

Should she break it off now or try to continue? She favored the latter because she truly loved being with Nolan and admitted to herself that she was in love with him and didn't want to lose him. She even toyed with the idea of asking Nolan to consider divorce, but she couldn't work up the nerve to suggest it.

In the meantime, during Sarah's absence in Shreveport, Nolan and Debbie continued to see each other. Although they each understood what had happened and that the result would lead to a change in their relationship, neither was prepared to deal with that eventuality. They still enjoyed their time together, including the intimacy.

Nolan, following a moment of such intimacy, said, "I do love you and wish I could spend the rest of my life in your embrace." "Well, Nolan, you'll have to make some decisions soon, if that's what you want."

But Nolan again reverted to his characteristic uncertainty and his inability to arrive at a decision, much less act on it, and he continued to delay making one.

Debbie's complex relationship with Nolan—her willingness to become involved with a married man—had strong roots that went back to her own childhood. She was the daughter of a single woman who, Debbie discovered, had had many clandestine relationships. While briefly married, one of those relationships had resulted in pregnancy, and Debbie was the product. Her mother was an alcoholic and drug abuser, who often left Debbie and her half sister alone for long stretches of time, sometimes even overnight, without supervision or adequate food. This was while Mother was "visiting a friend" or barhopping with her buddies.

Debbie never knew her biological father, and there was never a man in the house for any significant time who could possibly have served as a male role model. Debbie grew up desperate for love and compassion. When she began to mature sexually, it was only a short time before she searched for that compassion, and immediately she lost her virginity. She continued to seek relationships with men and came to realize that she didn't trust other women. She needed male companionship to satisfy her emotional as well as her sexual needs.

At the age of eighteen, Debbie met Jake, who was at least ten years older than her and who made all sorts of promises to her that never turned out as they had been presented. They ran away and moved to Atlanta, where Jake took a job as a night watchman. He had told her he was a college graduate and had held jobs in high finance. He said he had plenty of money put away for them both. None of it was true.

When Jake began drinking heavily, he also started to abuse Debbie physically. He also had sexual proclivities that Debbie abhorred. Finally, she had to flee, which she did in the middle of the night, without any extra clothing, money, or means of supporting herself. She went to a shelter in Atlanta and then made the very difficult decision to call her mother and beg her way back into her home.

Much later, while sharing her life story with Nolan, she told him, "I was a wreck. Calling my mother for help, after having run away without a word to her, was the ultimate act of defeatism. I considered suicide but decided that that was too easy of a way out. I would suck it up, get back on my feet, find a job, and try to make something of my life, if at all possible."

The next several years were difficult for her, but she managed to support herself and enrolled in nursing school. First, she earned her LVN degree but decided that she wanted to be an RN, so she went back to school for two more years. After she'd graduated near the top of her class, the director of nursing at the school had offered Debbie a staff position, which she'd gratefully accepted. It was the first time in her life that someone had sincerely wanted her to stay around.

But Debbie's success with men had remained nonexistent. She'd taken up with a fellow nursing student and had lived with him for two years. He turned out to be a womanizer.

When Debbie had returned home from a shift one evening and found him in bed with another woman, she told him, "If you are not out of this apartment within fifteen minutes, I am going to grab the meat cleaver and cut off your dick before I kill you!"

He was gone in ten minutes.

Debbie left that job and made her way to Chicago, where she was hired as an ICU nurse in the same hospital where Nolan was on staff.

Nolan was the first married man who'd gotten her attention. His professional demeanor as a physician, his rugged good looks, and his outward confidence (it took a while for her to discover his insecurities) had attracted her immediately. That attraction had led to the bathroom episode, which she had carefully concocted.

Their affair was everything she had hoped. Nolan proved to be attentive to her needs, emotionally very compassionate, and a good listener. Debbie felt she could tell him virtually anything and everything, and she did so. She would have liked for Nolan to have done the same but soon recognized that it was not in his personality to divulge his innermost thoughts. Debbie attributed this, in part, to the "male gene"—she believed that men had a much more difficult time expressing their feelings than women. Since Nolan never told Debbie much about his upbringing, she had no knowledge of the genesis of his insecurities or his inability to share his deepest emotions. So, Debbie was satisfied to serve as the instigator of most of their conversations.

Debbie also recognized that she had a jealous streak, likely the result of her bad history with men and also the lack of a stable male in her maturing years. Therefore, when she was finally able to develop a secure relationship with a man, she guarded it fiercely. She kept a close eye on Nolan, particularly when she saw other women giving him a lookover.

Debbie decided that, if Nolan showed a desire to continue, she would gladly do so. But if he was reticent, if he told her he was going to resurrect his marriage, then she would be understanding, although saddened, and they would go their separate ways. She understood that she was the home-wrecker, the woman responsible for encouraging Nolan's straying from his marriage. She had rationalized that by convincing herself that his marriage was already floundering.

There's no question another woman eventually will entice him into an affair, she had rationalized. *He has a lot to offer a woman, even though he's married. So it might as well be me.*

CHAPTER 17
Counseling

NOLAN AND SARAH DECIDED TO SEE A COUNSELOR WHO CAME highly recommended by the social services department in Sarah's hospital and was trusted by Sarah. The counselor, it turned out, had served a similar role with at least two of Sarah's nursing colleagues.

The first several meetings were "pro forma," obtaining the personal history of each, the details of their courtship, early marriage years, childbearing and raising—this of course resulted in the painful recollections surrounding Jenny's death. Subsequent meetings delved into their current status and relationship, including how and why Nolan had become unfaithful.

Sarah continued to have difficulty relating to their counselor, just as she had when seeking professional help following the loss of Jenny. She was just unable to fully open up and trust a stranger with her innermost thoughts. That was a significant impairment to their progressing in the analysis of their difficulties or in providing any solutions. When the counselor delved into Sarah's formative years— her relationships with her parents—Sarah rebelled.

"This is not about me and my failures in relationships. It's about my husband and his infidelity. I will not be made responsible for the failure of our marriage!"

Nolan was quiet, preferring to let Sarah and the counselor carry the ball. When Sarah refused to allow the counselor to question her about her childhood and teen years, however, he knew this wasn't going anywhere.

That finished off formal counseling for the time being. Sarah felt now that she was without any support, and she once again turned to her friends for assistance.

One of her best friends, Allison, whom Sarah had known and confided in for at least ten years, was particularly helpful. She was a listener who helped Sarah gain insight into her own mind, how she was registering with what had happened, and how she might be able to deal with Nolan.

During one of their discussions, Allison sipped her second glass of Chablis and told Sarah, "I knew—at least, I suspected—that Nolan was having an affair for some time."

Sarah expressed shock and dismay at that revelation. Allison tried to backtrack, but Sarah wasn't having any of it. She pushed Allison into describing exactly what she had heard.

"A friend and I saw Nolan and Debbie at a restaurant in Chicago several months ago," Allison finally said. "We watched them and could tell they were relating to each other in a manner that was not what one would expect from people who were just friends. In fact, she had her hand in his lap—in a way that I suspected what she was reaching for." Allison took another sip of her wine. "It was common knowledge that Nolan had an eye for other women. He was often seen talking to them in the hospital, away from the patient areas. Of course, that type of activity could have been appropriate in certain situations, but I was highly suspicious."

Sarah initially turned on her friend, demanding, "Why didn't you say something to me before now?"

"You are my best friend, and I didn't want to do anything that could be hurtful to you, even if it was related to your marriage. I'm deeply ashamed that I betrayed you, and I'm so sorry that this has happened to you."

Sarah needed further confirmation that what Allison had told her was true, so she met with a mutual friend of hers and Allison's.

Though initially reticent, that second friend confirmed that the rumors were true. "I too saw Nolan in a somewhat compromising situation with another woman—a nurse at the surgicenter where they both worked." When pressured, she told Sarah, "It involved a passionate embrace in a darkened corridor."

Sarah, now completely distraught, took a couple of days off work, locked herself in her room, and avoided contact with Nolan—and, unfortunately, with James as well. When she had had enough time to make a decision and put together a plan, she emerged from her cocoon. She knew that enacting her plan, a divorce, would take time. In the meantime, she would continue as before— with raising James; with nursing; and with being a wife to Nolan, but in a manner best described as platonic.

CHAPTER 18
Money and the Practice of Medicine

THE SURGICENTER CONTINUED TO THRIVE. NOLAN AND HIS partners were earning a substantial amount of money, above and beyond what they earned for their surgical procedures. The center was profitable and able to make income distributions to its investors. Other physicians who were not surgeons but had invested in the center were also benefactors of the center's success, in part because they referred patients to the center for surgery, rather than to the hospital. In some states, this might have been judged as illegal, a form of self-referral for financial gain, but not in Illinois.4

For an orthopedist who needs to view a patient's healing fracture with an X-ray, having an X-ray machine in the office is more efficient and convenient for the patient than sending the patient to a radiologist's office or a hospital for the same X-ray. The fact that the orthopedist collects an additional fee for the X-ray is generally seen as reasonable. The same principle could just as reasonably be applied to the aforementioned fictitious cardiologist. Why should the patient go to another imaging center for the test if the cardiologist has the same equipment in his office? Whether or not the cardiologist had the same training and level of expertise as the nuclear medicine specialist is the subject of considerable medical controversy.

It became cloudier when, for instance, the orthopedist sees a patient with a knee problem and wants to do an MRI. Orthopedists had little training in performing and interpreting MRI studies, but they often argue that they should be able to own an MRI unit and refer their patients for a study. The cost and remuneration for MRIs is substantial. Is it possible that the orthopedist is "gaming the system"—that an MRI is not really necessary for proper decisionmaking regarding the patient? Could the substantial fee the orthopedist would collect from the MRI affect the decision to have it performed on his or her patient? Does the orthopedist have the advanced training required to properly perform and interpret an MRI? Those and other similar situations speaks to the heart of selfreferral. Regardless of one's opinion, it is a fact that, from a pure cost standpoint, studies have shown that self-referral added substantial cost to health care in the United States.5

In addition to filing the lawsuit, the hospitals fought back in other ways. They wrote letters to newspapers, decrying what the physicians were doing, saying it was negatively affecting the hospitals and, indirectly, the entire medical community. They pointed out that poorer people, those without adequate insurance coverage, were particularly at risk, since the center did nothing to assist them and even turned away many who were unable to pay the full fare. The administrators and members of the board of directors of the hospitals also lobbied politicians, in particular the Chicago aldermen who served on the City of Chicago Council. They also lobbied at the state of Illinois level, attempting to get legislation passed that would prohibit independent centers from participating in Medicare and Medicaid funding.

Although there was no immediate effect—no reduction of utilization or payments to the center—the publicity was distinctly negative. The surgicenter management was concerned about the possible longterm effects of the lobbying. In an attempt to counter the hospitals' charges, the center managers hired a public relations company to write letters to the newspapers and politicians, pointing out how beneficial the new center was as an additional point of service in the community.

After a year's operational time, due to all the controversy and, in particular, the impending lawsuit, a rift developed within Nolan's surgical partnership. Of the fifteen senior partners, eight supported the center and its activity (they were all investors), and seven wanted to separate from it. Partnership meetings were intense, sometimes angry, with invectives spilling out from both sides.

The center's supporters would say such things to the increasinglydisenchanted physicians as, "You knew from the very beginning that the center would be controversial and that the hospitals would be against it. Why in hell didn't you speak out then? How naive can you be?"

One doctor/investor who had become disenchanted with the surgicenter said, "Yes, we knew that, but we didn't expect that the center's investors would be concerned only with the financial bottom line. We expected, maybe naively, that it would at least attempt to be stewards of the community and to offer to discount some care to those less fortunate, who had less insurance coverage. Was that too much to expect?"

Another supporter of the center responded, "Yes, you are naive. You cannot expect for an investor, in this or any other financial endeavor, to go out of pocket and support people who cannot afford a provided service. Where would that stop? Are we expected to underwrite health care costs for the entire community, maybe even for the entire country?"

The dilemma, both existential and practical, became manifest as an overwhelming concern with the lawsuit. Their attorneys judged they had a fifty-fifty likelihood of succeeding, and this was too much for some of the partners. They demanded that the partnership dissolve, thus freeing them to resume practice solely at the hospital; they believed that action would likely result in their dismissal from the lawsuit.

Nolan, Burt, and a couple of their colleagues were bitterly opposed to dissolution. They feared that would damage the group, collectively and individually, and make them pariahs in the medical and general communities.

Nolan thought back to the reasons he'd gone into medicine in the first place. He was extremely distressed. *How did I get into this mess in the first place? he asked himself. Was it greed or just ignorance?*

He hadn't spent much time in his early days of practice figuring out how he could earn more money; he and Sarah had long ago decided that money wouldn't be the driving force of his career. But here he was, and he no longer had Sarah at his side for input and counsel. He sorely missed her for that.

At a preliminary hearing, a judge announced a stay order, which would permit the hospitals to suspend any physician who was a certified investor in the surgicenter until a final legal decision had been made. That resulted in even more havoc among the investors, forcing them to choose, even if legally only temporarily, between the hospitals and the surgicenter for their livelihoods. After much soulsearching and discussions with the lawyers and accountants, Nolan decided to remain with the surgicenter. In effect, that meant he and his similarly minded colleagues would be leaving the surgical partnership, as well as resigning from the hospital medical staff.

Dissolution proceedings commenced. A group of talented, committed physician surgeons, who had served the community faithfully for more than twenty-five years, was finished as a medical entity.

Two weeks later, two hospitals notified Nolan that his surgical and admitting privileges had been suspended and that he had been removed from all committees on which he was serving.

CHAPTER 19
Debbie, with Demands

DEBBIE WAS BEYOND EXASPERATED. SHE HAD TRIED TO TALK with Nolan to find out what he was planning to do with his life and whether it would involve her. But she could not get him to commit to anything; he refused to give her straight answers.

"Nolan, you have to make some decisions. I'm not trying to pressure you. But do you plan on returning to Sarah and making amends, or is it over for the two of you?"

"I don't know," he said. "You know she found out about us, about me—and likely other more minor incidents—and she said that she is strongly considering a divorce."

"Strongly considering? What does that mean? Did she say it to you that way?"

"Not exactly, but the meaning was clear. She hasn't used the word divorce yet."

"You are a fool," Debbie snapped. "If a woman wants a divorce, she will tell you so in no uncertain terms. You have to decide what you want and then get on with your life. Make a decision, for God's sake!"

But Nolan didn't take Debbie's advice. He strung Debbie along and continued to try to have it both ways—to work on his marriage with the hope of it continuing and to be able to keep her as a mistress. That wasn't going to work for Debbie. She couldn't see herself continuing to sneak around with Nolan, knowing that his wife would again find out eventually. Debbie wasn't about to go through the same trauma a second time.

She finally gave Nolan the ultimatum that she had avoided for so long: "Either you obtain a divorce, or you reconcile with Sarah. If you do the latter, then I will understand, and we will end this, once and for all." With that, she gently but firmly escorted him out of her apartment.

She had trouble believing what had happened to her yet again— another relationship gone to hell. *Why am I unable to find someone to share my life without so much drama?*

Debbie was an intelligent woman, but she was too directly involved to step back and reflect on that rhetorical question. That she was the one responsible for ending Nolan's marriage didn't occur to her either; or it was more likely the case that she didn't want to accept it. Regardless, she made a solemn vow that she would live up to her promise to Nolan—she would be gone if he decided to stay with Sarah.

CHAPTER 20
Sarah, Decisive

ONCE SARAH MADE HER DECISION, IT WAS FULL SPEED AHEAD. "I can't remain married to you," she told him. "You have violated my trust repeatedly and have not shown that you're willing to cease your infidelities and work on our marriage. I'm moving out of here and taking James with me. We'll remain in Chicago so that you can spend time with your son."

Nolan's reaction was surprisingly calm. It was as if he knew what was coming and had prepared for her announcement. He expressed only mild remorse, not even raising a ruckus regarding custody of James.

"Don't you feel at all bad about not being able to live with your son?" Sarah asked.

"You are a much better, much more devoted parent than I am or ever will be," he said. "Besides, with the demands of my practice and the pending lawsuit, I would have little time to spend with James anyhow. It's best if he lives with you, and I'll see him whenever possible."

Sarah was rendered speechless by Nolan's total lack of emotion and his acceptance of the loss of his family. His using his career and questionable decision-making with the surgicenter as an excuse to desert his family was incredible to her. She looked at Nolan for a brief moment and left the room.

Over the course of several days, Sarah met with a lawyer and an accountant to assess her financial situation. She found a small two-bedroom apartment in the neighborhood so that James could remain in the same school, and she somehow continued working as well. She tearfully told her nurse supervisor, "I'll need to work almost full-time, now that I'm on my own."

"The hospital is completely satisfied with you as a nurse," her boss said. "We'll be glad to have you, as much as you're able to manage."

When Sarah called her parents to tell them what was happening, she finally broke down and cried. She had told herself that she could control her emotions, but this time, that was not possible. It was the first time in her adult life that she had cried on the telephone—the first time that she had allowed herself to display her emotions so openly to her mother.

Her parents were consoling.

"Is there anything we can do immediately?" her mother asked.

"We can come to Chicago to help you," her father added.

But Sarah refused their offer. She felt that would impede her recovery, rather than assist with it.

Sarah reflected on the situation. *It was difficult enough for me to divulge the breakup of my marriage to my parents, she thought. I can't bear the thought of having them around constantly, seeing my grief and humiliation.*

Sarah's siblings were extremely supportive.

Her older sister, Winnie, said, "I demand that you allow me to visit you. I know you would do it for me. I'll be on a plane for Chicago tomorrow."

CHAPTER 21
Young James

WITH ALL THAT NOLAN HAD TO DEAL WITH AFTER SARAH moved out, the most difficult part was that James was no longer living under his roof. Nolan came to realize that he had taken his son for granted. He hadn't spent the time with James he had told himself he would, especially after Jenny's death.

Like so many young boys, James idolized sports stars. He loved the Chicago Cubs, in part because Wrigley Field was only a few miles from his home. His family would pass by it frequently. He had never been to a game but was thrilled with the stories his father told him of players such as Billy Williams; Ron Santo; and "Mr. Cub," Ernie Banks. Nolan frequently quoted Ernie's famous saying, "It's a beautiful day; let's play two!"

When Nolan surprised James one summer day with tickets to an upcoming Cubs / Red Sox game, James was ecstatic. He barely slept for the three days prior to the game, and he kept his baseball glove in his bed, next to his pillow. When game day came and they reached their seats behind third base and James could hear the ballplayers talking among themselves during batting practice, he was in heaven.

Even during the game, which turned into a pitching duel—Nolan was hoping it would be a slugfest, knowing that kids would rather watch home runs than a screwball thrown for a called strike three— James was attentive for much of the game. Eventually, though, he began paying more attention to the hot dogs and Cokes that Nolan brought to their seats about every third inning, the usual outcome for a youngster during a long game.

Following the game, when Nolan took James home to his mother, he stayed to tuck his tired, half-asleep son into bed. As he did so, James asked, "Why can't we all live together like we used to?"

Nolan again tried to explain the circumstances, saying, "Your mother and I are trying to sort some things out, and that means we need to live separately for now. We both love you dearly. We will always be here for you, no matter what else happens." In a lastditch effort to mollify James, he added, "I promise I'll take you to another ball game very soon."

He knew Sarah had also been trying to explain things to James, but the concept was beyond the understanding of a young child, who only wanted both his parents to be with him in their shared home.

Nolan knew that the Burkett family's situation was not unique. Separation and divorce had become a part of the American cultural scene and was increasing consistently. Children suffered the consequences more severely than did their parents, as the children had virtually no control over the events or eventual outcome. The psychological toll was enormous and almost certainly accounted for a major portion of teenage rebellion, drug and alcohol abuse, and poor choices in companionship (and the often-resultant pregnancy). Would James be one who suffered from his parents' inability to maintain an intact family? No one could predict that, but the odds were certainly turning against him.

After a short rest, Nolan phoned Debbie. "I need to see you and to be with you. The last several weeks have been crazy, and it's a certainty that I'll be divorced very soon. Please tell me that you love and need me as much as I do you."

Debbie was reserved and noncommittal, but she did consent to letting him come to her apartment.

CHAPTER 22
Nolan, at a Crossroad

NOLAN AND SARAH'S DIVORCE WAS FINALIZED IN ABOUT SIX months. The settlement was surprisingly amicable and fair. Sarah and Nolan decided not to fight it out for every dollar, knowing that, in those circumstances, it is primarily the lawyers who win. Besides, neither wanted James to be subjected to the endless arguments and emotional outbursts that would have resulted from a contentious divorce.

Nolan missed the complex surgical cases he had previously performed in the hospital. He felt that, if his absence from the operating room continued, his surgical skills would suffer, possibly irreparably. He decided to apply to another hospital, several miles distant from home, in order to gain access to a hospital operating room. The problem was he had no referrals for that hospital. Almost all his referring physicians, as well as the vast majority of patients, did not want to leave the immediate area for medical practice and care. Very few cases resulted from his new staff membership.

He had given up his clinical instructorship at the university as well, and he missed the teaching aspect of medicine; he missed "rounding" with the eager young residents and nurses who were always part of those programs. When he applied to yet another Chicago university in hopes of regaining what he had given up, he was told that, in addition to making hospital rounds and scrubbing into surgery with the residents, he would be expected to give formal classroom instruction at least twice a month. He had no interest in doing that, so he withdrew his application.

He told Debbie, "Teaching young physicians the basics of surgical practice, how to interview a patient, and what the landmarks for an abdominal incision are would bore me to tears in a few short days."

Nolan's affair with Debbie continued, but some of the previous passion had dissipated. It was difficult to say whether that was the result of their not knowing what their future together would be. Regardless, it had changed, and not for the better.

When Nolan suggested to Debbie that, now that he was divorced, they could consider living together, she answered, "No. I want to be able to remain unattached." And as a further surprise to Nolan, she told him, "If I choose to have a relationship with another man, I want to be free to do so."

Nolan was surprised and crushed by this announcement. "You told me before that I was the only man with whom you wanted to spend your life."

"Yes, I did. But I've had a lot of time to think on this, and I'm less sure about that now. My relationships with men, as you know, have not been exactly exemplary. I'd like to think that, if I try to begin another one, it will have a chance of being successful."

"I really think that I can be that man, Debbie. I've learned a lot over the years. One of the things I've learned is to not take any relationship for granted. I promise you I will never do that with you."

Debbie listened to his impassioned pleas but remained steadfast. She was not ready to commit.

In addition to the problems in his relationship with Debbie, Nolan was suffering from ennui, a combination of anxiety and boredom. The only diversions from work were his occasional nights out for music or meals with friends and the less-than-frequent time with James. He and James enjoyed being together, particularly when it involved a ball game or a visit to the zoo, aquarium, or amusement park. Otherwise, his evenings were rather quiet, especially if Debbie was not available.

His next venture was to buy a sports car. Nolan had delayed this purchase while married, as Sarah frowned on such an "ostentatious possession," as she called it. Now, it was different. He decided on a Porsche roadster. Initially, he wanted a red or yellow one but settled for black, a little less conspicuous.

The car was beautiful, it was extremely fast and purred like a very large cat. Driving it in the city was difficult. He couldn't really get it moving, so he would take long drives toward neighboring Wisconsin or southern Illinois in order to open it up. The thrill was palpable while the drive lasted, but when he returned home, he almost immediately relapsed into a mood of passivity and remorse.

Several weeks later, Nolan was in a neighborhood grocery market when a middle-aged woman approached him in line. "I know you. You're Dr. Burkett, the surgeon. I used to work with you as a surgical nurse in the hospital. My name is Becky."

"Hi, Becky. Yes, I remember you. You were always so quick and accurate with the surgical instruments. I never had to name one of them for you. Your anticipatory skills were that good!"

They chatted for a couple of minutes, and then Becky said, "Dr. Burkett, I left the hospital to become a nurse at the Chicago Free Clinic on State Street. It was the best thing I ever did. Would you ever consider visiting the clinic to see what it does for people in Chicago?"

Nolan was rendered speechless. It was the first time in a long while that someone had asked him to do something different and positive. It took a moment for Becky's remarks to sink in before he answered, "I'd be delighted to do that. Please give me the contact information, and I'll get right on it. And please call me Nolan. We're no longer in a professional situation."

"Thank you, Nolan. Here's one of their cards. When you call, please mention my name and ask that they invite you to visit the clinic, preferably when I'm scheduled to work."

CHAPTER 23
Reinvigoration

WHEN NOLAN CALLED THE CHICAGO FREE CLINIC A FEW days later, an excited Becky arranged for Nolan to tour the facility with the head of the clinic, a retired medical internist named John DeFranco. Dr. DeFranco had been with the clinic since its inception in the 1980s —it was the third in the nation to be established, following those in San Francisco and New York. John told Nolan that the clinic serviced the central and southern portions of the city primarily, with a few patients coming from as far away as Cicero, Illinois. The clinic generally saw forty to fifty patients per day, six days a week.

Occasionally, a private hospital agreed to support a small portion of the clinic's needs. Since there was almost no income generated from its patients (insurance companies did not recognize the free clinics as a reimbursable medical facility), the clinic relied on volunteer staffing; gifts from a few Chicago businesses; individual contributions; and, of late, a few grants from the state of Illinois. In addition, the clinic was in the midst of negotiating with Chicago's medical universities for shared services and a modicum of financial support.

Dr. DeFranco told Nolan, "We see an incredible variety of medical situations at the clinic. They range from the 'purely internal medical,' such as diabetic ketoacidosis (diabetes out of control), malignant hypertension, and pneumonia to gynecological and urinary tract disorders that are often very serious. Sometimes we see surgical cases such as diverticulitis and appendicitis that we have to refer to our surrounding hospitals."

Nolan told Dr. DeFranco that he'd had similar experiences as a student while rotating through the San Francisco Free Clinic. "I never dreamed that I might relive that experience! But now, I'm a thoracic surgeon who has been away from general medical practice for many years. I'm not sure I'm ready or able to handle those not-surgical situations you describe."

Dr. DeFranco wasn't having any of that, telling Nolan, "I've seen your application. Any surgeon with your training and experience would be a welcome addition to our staff."

Nolan was impressed with the facility. It was clean and brightly lit and painted—a very welcoming though small building that was well maintained. The staff he met that day was cheerful, almost to the point of exuberance. And even though some of the equipment was a little bit dated and obviously had been donated in a previously used condition, it was spotless and certainly functional. In fact, Nolan thought the gynecological exam table was better than what he had used during his San Francisco General Hospital days.

Nolan told Dr. DeFranco and Becky that he would like to attend at the clinic for a couple of days during the following month to see how he would fit in. He was accepted immediately and given a temporary staff appointment and even an identification badge that had been prepared in anticipation of his visit. They were ready for him!

On his first day at the clinic—a Saturday following a hectic week of private practice—Nolan showed up for work at 7:00 a.m. His very first patient was a very young woman, who told the clinical nurse assigned to her, "I have a very foul discharge coming from my vagina."

After a short history (including a somewhat halting inquiry into the patient's recent sexual relations), an examination revealed that the patient had discharge and evidence of cervicitis (inflammation of the cervix, commonly related to venereal disease). Nolan obtained a culture of the discharge and prescribed an antibiotic that hopefully would be beneficial. He also counseled the patient on the absolute necessity of refraining from sexual activity for at least two weeks and the use of condoms following that time.

After the patient left the clinic, Nolan took the nurse aside and asked, "How do you think I did? That was the first patient with a venereal disease I've attended in more than fifteen years."

The nurse smiled and said to Nolan, "If every patient had access to physicians with your level of competency and concern, the city of Chicago would be disease-free in a few months!" It was a bit of an overstatement, but Nolan felt gratified and was ready to see another patient.

By the end of his shift—and another, two weeks later— Nolan had seen about twenty-five patients. All had relatively mild problems— some with bladder or throat infections, one with pneumonia that showed on a chest X-ray, and several with skin conditions that befuddled Nolan; he had last seen a patient with a dermatological condition as a fourth-year medical student, and he never had enjoyed dermatology. The only serious situation was that of a young man who came in with a fever and complaints of severe abdominal pain. Nolan's exam strongly suggested that the patient had appendicitis, possibly to the point of rupture and, thus, lifethreatening. He called one of the university hospitals, got through to a surgical resident, and arranged for the patient to be transferred to the hospital by ambulance. (Nolan took personal financial responsibility for the ambulance.)

The next day, the surgeon called Nolan and told him that, indeed, the patient did have appendicitis; he had undergone surgery and was recovering satisfactorily.

Nolan thanked the surgeon and invited him to come to the clinic for a visit and tour.

The surgeon declined. "My position as a staff resident leaves very little time for extra responsibilities."

Nolan understood that very well.

Debbie hadn't seen Nolan so excited or positive in a long time. When he arrived at her apartment several weeks after his initial work at the free clinic, Nolan immediately began describing the clinic to her and told her of some of the patients he had seen and, hopefully, helped. He could use medical jargon with Debbie in describing some of the illnesses and the potential serious conditions, including the case of appendicitis. He also told her of another patient who'd turned out to have a large intra-abdominal abscess; that patient had also required immediate hospitalization and surgery and was recovering.

Debbie sensed that Nolan was enthusiastic, in part because he had reclaimed some of his earlier personal satisfaction that came from making a difference in peoples' lives. He'd been doing that in private practice as well, but the free clinic patients were both truly in need and extremely appreciative of the care that was provided, at virtually no personal cost to them.

Nolan told Debbie, "I haven't had that level of satisfaction as a physician since my days at the San Francisco Free Clinic."

Debbie was once again a terrific listener and sounding board for Nolan. But this time, she also had a suggestion for him. "Why don't you approach your partners, particularly the ones at the surgicenter, and ask them to donate some time, services, and equipment to the free clinic? Some of them would likely react similarly to how you have. It would be very good community service to Chicago and likely good public relations for the surgicenter."

After mulling over Debbie's suggestion, Nolan's response was predictable. "There's no way in hell those guys would be willing to sacrifice their time or to take any financial risk, which could be considerable for them personally, as well as for the surgicenter. I just don't think that it would work."

But Nolan thought more about Debbie's suggestion. Later that evening he said, "I still don't think it will happen, but I'm willing to give it a try. Maybe I'll arrange a meeting with a few of the docs to see if there's any interest."

After that, Nolan put on a Beethoven sonata CD, opened a bottle of wine, and proceeded to seduce Debbie in a manner that he hadn't done for some time.

Following a very enjoyable experience for each, Debbie, somewhat breathlessly, managed to say, "If I had known that your mood and emotions would improve so dramatically following a reassessment of your medical career, I would have suggested some of those changes much earlier!"

CHAPTER 24
The Proposal

NOLAN MADE AN INFORMAL PRESENTATION TO TWO OF HIS most trusted partners over dinner the following week. One of those partners was Burt, who had remained Nolan's friend as well as surgical colleague.

Nolan told them what he'd been doing at the free clinic over the recent months. "I plan to continue and possibly even increase my volunteer time," he said. "And I'm in the process of recruiting other medical personnel—physicians, nurses, lab, and radiology technologists—to volunteer as well." Then Nolan outlined his (actually, Debbie's) idea that maybe the surgicenter could be involved. "Would either of you have any personal interest in participating? Do you think that other members of the surgicenter ownership would be open to the idea?"

As Nolan had anticipated, their initial reaction was that of total surprise, bordering on shock. Neither had any idea of what Nolan had been doing at the free clinic; one of them didn't even know that the clinic existed. And though they hemmed and hawed about possibly considering personal involvement—maybe an occasional day per month—as a volunteer, they were much more skeptical in regard to getting the surgicenter into the mix.

They were good friends as well as Nolan's colleagues, however, so they did agree to at least support a more formal meeting and presentation to some of the other partners.

Nolan expressed his appreciation for that level of commitment, telling them, "I promise that I'll do all the legwork, including setting up the meeting, inviting our colleagues, and preparing a written and verbal plan for how the venture might be arranged. I'll even spring for a small luncheon as further enticement!"

Nolan realized he was taking on a significant task that would further stretch his own time management. That was already a problem; his time at the clinic was impacting, among other things, the time he was trying to spend with James.

"Debbie, this is probably a mistake. I don't think any of them are going to go for it, and it will probably result in my being ostracized from the group."

"Well, you'll never know for sure unless you make the attempt. I understand your concern. And believe me, I also understand that decision-making has always been difficult for you. But I have confidence in you. I know you can present yourself well and honestly. Just give it your best effort, and let's see what happens."

The meeting was unlike anything Nolan had attended or arranged before. He invited thirty-five of the fifty investors in the surgicenter; he was convinced that the remainder would be strongly opposed to any type of participation.

For openers, he asked Dr. John DeFranco, the internist administrator of the free clinic, to open the meeting and to briefly describe both its history and current status. Then, an experienced health insurance executive, who Nolan he had come to know during his role in setting up the surgicenter, addressed the group. That executive, somewhat surprisingly to Nolan, proposed that some health insurance companies might recognize the financial legitimacy of the free clinic, in large part because medical expenses for patients at such a clinic would likely compare favorably to those for standard hospitals and clinics.

Nolan noticed that several physicians paid close attention to those remarks.

Following Nolan's talk, he related his personal satisfaction with providing care to the indigent population of Chicago and his heightened awareness of their medical needs. Following that, there was a question-and-answer period. Originally scheduled to last twenty-five minutes, the session lasted for over an hour. Only the already-delayed luncheon and other personal commitments of the doctors kept it from lasting longer.

When the meeting concluded, several physicians approached Nolan and congratulated him on the meeting. Several made it clear that, although they were still skeptical as to whether an alliance between the free clinic and the surgicenter should happen, they were eager and willing to delve into it more closely. Several others left the meeting abruptly, even forgoing the luncheon, obviously not pleased with any of what had transpired.

Nolan was asked to set up yet another meeting, this time to include legal and accounting consultants, some of whom had been involved with the surgicenter from its inception. Nolan agreed to do so. He realized yet again that, if anything positive was to come of all this, it was on his shoulders to get it done.

The follow-up meeting was, somewhat predictably, more contentious and problematic. To start, the accountants and lawyers who were asked to weigh in on the project were dubious. Conservative by nature, training, and experience, they warned the physicians against participating in the venture. While most of their admonitions consisted of the usual warnings about potential financial encumberment and possible loss, they had other concerns as well. Particularly noted was malpractice insurance. Malpractice insurance had been a bugaboo for physicians in the United States for decades, relating in large measure to a propensity for high-cost malpractice suits; the lawyers who specialized in pursuing them; and, in some states (including Illinois), the lack of liability limits for adverse judgments. (See "Conclusion")

All of this could be argued from the other side as well, mainly the need to recompense patients who had suffered from verifiable malpractice and malfeasance.

The risks for the surgicenter could be substantial, they stated emphatically. The lawyers could not assure the physicians that financial protection—insurance coverage, both for the surgicenter as well as for them as individuals—could be obtained.

The accountants raised the question of how such a partnership between the surgicenter and a nonprofit free clinic could even be established. There was no known precedent or model to use, and most of the physician investors were not keen on being a trial balloon.

Finally, a vote of the executive committee of the surgicenter was taken. The committee voted to recommend to the general partnership that the surgicenter should not be formally tied to the free clinic. However, they did state that they would encourage individual physicians and others associated with the surgicenter, including nurses, aides, and technologists, to volunteer to serve in the clinic on their own time. They made it clear that they were impressed with all that the clinic was doing for the community, and they would support it and consider financial grants-in-aid, donations of equipment, and other means that might be developed. The committee also congratulated Nolan for his efforts.

Nolan was not surprised by the decision. After all, he knew his associates, and he knew that physicians were generally risk-averse. Even those who were supportive of the venture had expressed reservations about the wisdom of involving the surgicenter, legally, with the free clinic.

At the end of the last meeting, however, several physicians and nurses congratulated Nolan and volunteered on the spot to serve the free clinic. He was equally surprised and appreciative. He felt that his efforts, though not completely rewarded, were also not in vain.

Burt told him, "You've got balls, Nolan, to go before a medical group and propose something so contrary to its training and manner of practicing medicine. I've got to hand it to you for making the effort, even if it comes to naught."

"Thank you, Burt, for the backhanded compliment! I'm going to try to prove you wrong about the success of my efforts to involve the medical community with the free clinic."

Debbie was even less surprised by the decision. As a nurse, she had come to expect that many physicians were more interested in their own financial gain than in the welfare of society as a whole. She admitted that she was a cynic but also said, "I'm a realist as well." And she applauded Nolan's willingness to put his reputation on the line, his stubborn resolve to attempt to advance the project, and his renewed belief in a physician's role in providing care for the less fortunate. Debbie made her admiration of Nolan known repeatedly over the following weeks and months and volunteered some of her time for the free clinic. She was definitely reassessing her personal opinions in regard to Nolan and their possible future together.

"Nolan, I'm so proud of you! It took real guts to put yourself, your reputation, and your career on the line in front of all those physicians. And you can take a little pride in your efforts as well. It's time that you acknowledge yourself for a change."

CHAPTER 25
Going Forward

NOLAN CONTINUED AS HE HAD BEFORE. HE SPENT MOST OF HIS time with patients at the surgicenter, but he also continued to attend at one of the other major hospitals. His role with the free clinic continued and even increased, as he was also given some administrative responsibilities, which included being asked to raise funds in the community and from several medical societies. He also helped to prepare applications for state and even federal grants, including research funds for investigation of HIV-related diseases. That seemed a natural to Nolan, what with the unfortunate abundance of AIDS patients being attended to at the clinic.

On one Saturday morning, while working at the clinic, Nolan was summoned in emergency fashion to one of the waiting rooms. There, Dr. DeFranco was sitting slumped in a chair, breathing rapidly, and having difficulty speaking. After a rapid assessment, Nolan called the paramedics and had Dr. DeFranco taken to the local hospital. Within a few hours, it was determined that the doctor had suffered a significant stroke. Following a few days in the hospital he partially recovered, but his days attending the free clinic were likely over, at least for the short run.

The free clinic staff was in shock. Dr. DeFranco had been the heart and soul of the clinic since its founding fifteen years ago. Most of the staff had never even considered what would happen when he was gone. At an emergency staff meeting, several staff members, including a few of Nolan's associates and other physicians and nurses who knew him, asked Nolan if he would consider assuming the role as head of the clinic.

Nolan, also recovering from the loss of Dr. DeFranco from the clinic, was taken aback by the offer and was unsure how to answer. He expressed his gratitude to the group for their confidence in him and requested a few days to think it over.

Nolan felt he was at a crossroads in his career, and he was ambivalent. On one hand, he had a desire to serve the clinic, but that would require a significant increase in his time and efforts. He had a renewed sense of worth when he worked there, and he didn't want to lose it. On the other hand, he knew he would suffer a significant decrease in his income as a result of less time available for private practice and that his surgical skills would inevitably suffer as well. He knew that, if he took the clinic job full-time, he would never perform the complicated procedures for which he was trained and had been performing for many years.

Nolan had the good sense to include Debbie in the decision-making process. He had learned to trust her judgment, which he regarded as at least equal in value to his own. He also wondered what might have happened with his marriage to Sarah if he had trusted her in that same fashion, but it was too late for that.

Debbie, again composed and organized, asked Nolan to prepare a list of personal values. She asked him, "What are the most and least important aspects of your life, including your family, your medical career, your material possessions, and your ultimate goals in life?"

It was a daunting challenge, but Nolan took it on.

Two weeks later Nolan asked to meet with several members of the free clinic—physicians, nurses, and heads of ancillary services—to present his personal decision. He also included Burt Scott, who remained his closest medical confidant. And he asked Debbie to be present during the meeting as well.

A week later, a formal announcement was made to the public that Nolan Burkett had been named the chief administrator and medical director for the Chicago Free Clinic. The Chicago Tribune placed the action on page one of its city section. The Chicago Surgical Society and several of Chicago's university centers published the news as well. Nolan's transformation was complete.

On the eve of the third anniversary of his daughter, Jenny's, death, Nolan called Sarah and asked if she would consider bringing James to join him on a visit to the cemetery where Jenny was buried. Sarah said, "Yes, I will."

They arrived almost simultaneously that morning, James with his new puppy in tow. James had named the puppy Buddy, which happened, not by coincidence, to be the name that Nolan often used when addressing James.

As they stood beside Jenny's grave—James between his parents, holding Buddy—James said, "Mommy, Daddy, I wish that Jenny was here with me to hold and play with Buddy. She would like him."

Nolan cautiously reached out and put his arm around Sarah's shoulder, and they both wept quietly.

CHAPTER 26
Finale

DURING THE COURSE OF THE NEXT SIX MONTHS, NOLAN WAS AS busy as he had ever been, including during his residency days. He had recruited a dozen staff members, including physicians, nurses, and technicians. He had raised almost $150,000 from various philanthropies in Chicago, and he'd secured a grant of $100,000 from his surgicenter. Using these funds, Nolan hired a full-time clinical manager, a nurse supervisor, and several more ancillary persons who would help the clinic to run more efficiently. Two of the universities in Chicago became affiliated with the clinic and planned to have family practice residents rotate through the clinic on a scheduled basis. And one of them formalized a clinical research partnership for AIDS research, as he had hoped.

Nolan also became a part-time surgical associate at one of the university hospitals. This position was an entry-level professional one but included a modest stipend and the right to see some private patients as well.

As Nolan evaluated his time allocation and financial situation, he realized something had to give. He couldn't continue with all he had been doing, in addition to managing his increasing responsibilities at the free clinic. He decided he would sell his partnership share in the surgicenter. Because the surgicenter had become so successful (each share had at least tripled in value), it was not difficult to find a buyer; physician investors were champing at the bit to join it.

With these funds, as well as the income from his university-based surgical practice, Nolan believed he could make do. It might require some lifestyle changes, but he had decided, with Debbie's encouragement, that a more modest lifestyle would be a very good idea.

And he sold the Porsche.

Conclusion

I HAVE TOLD NOLAN'S STORY IN THE THIRD PERSON, THE STYLE that most novelists use to tell the story of a fictional character, but I have chosen to write the conclusion in the first person. My reasons for doing so will become clear in short order.

Let me begin with the positive. I know of no profession or career that offers as many opportunities to make a difference in peoples' lives as does a medical career. Our society relies on high-quality medical care and generally venerates all those who take part (physicians, dentists, nurses, technologists, pharmacists, and ancillary service personnel of all types) in providing that care. The financial rewards for physicians, at least in the United States, are significant, enough to enable most to live comfortably, raise a family, and prepare for a retirement free of worry and stress. More on that later on.

For the vast majority of aspiring physicians who began, as did I, with a strong appreciation for and interest in the biological sciences, medicine is a terrific career choice. There are other careers available in the biological sciences, including research, education/teaching, and the world of technological and pharmaceutical development, to name but a few. But for those like me who enjoy the opportunity to interact with people and to occasionally make a significant difference in each of their lives, a career in medicine is where it's at.

Medicine is also intellectually stimulating. In my own field of radiology, the development and changes that have occurred over the last five decades are truly incredible. When I was in training in the 1970s, ultrasound was in its infancy. Computed tomography, arguably the most significant diagnostic innovation since Conrad Roentgen's discovery of the X-ray, was not available. (Some readers might want to choose from several biographies concerning the development of CT by Godfrey Hounsfield of EMI Corporation, coincidentally the same company that signed the Beatles and owned their song list for many years). Nuclear medicine with positron imaging was also unheard of. And in the 1990s, the development of magnetic resonance imaging, or MRI, with its unique method of body imaging that doesn't depend on radiation and its resultant damaging effects on living tissue, was revolutionary.

Many other medical disciplines of which I have been either a participant or merely an envious observer have made similarly incredible advances. Society has benefitted from those advances in the fields of genetics; immunology; chemotherapy; Gamma Knife, microscopic and robotic surgery; interventional radiologic procedures, including stents for cardiac, neurological, and extremity vascular obstruction; and endoscopy for surgery and diagnostic examinations alike. These are but a few of the myriad tests and procedures that have truly changed the science and art of medicine. And, they've provided intellectual stimulation and direct participation for virtually everyone who has practiced medicine since the 1960s.

Does the medical field attract the small number of true geniuses in our society? Can it compete with the world of physics to beckon the future Einsteins and Newtons; provide stimulus for the technological and marketing geniuses like Steve Jobs and Bill Gates; or the business entrepreneurs and inventors, such as Edison, Franklin, Ford, and Rockefeller? I would argue that it can because it has for years—by way of examples, Louis Pasteur with pasteurization, Salk with the polio vaccine, Madame

Curie with radium, Fleming with penicillin, and a host of other luminaries who have been responsible for saving countless millions of lives and serve as beacons for those few persons who will reach the pinnacle of human endeavor. They are few in number, to be sure, but for all who strive to reach the top, those and other great scientists serve as models for young scientists to guide them in their future endeavors.

Philosophers and authors over the centuries have used various aspects of the world of medicine on which to ascribe their teaching and storytelling, usually in a positive light. Hippocrates was the father of medicine in the fifth century BCE, and the Hippocratic oath is still recited by most medical school students at their commencements. The physician-turned-author Somerset Maugham, in *Of Human Bondage,* wrote of the perils but also the worthiness of the medical profession. The book *The Brothers Mayo* serves as an example of the twentieth century's efforts to establish scientifically sound methods for the practice of medicine. Sinclair Lewis's book *Arrowsmith* creates a hero, though not without faults, out of a country physician who strives to provide the best possible care for his patients. Other examples of enlightened behavior serve as templates for future medical professionals as they make their way in a world that desperately needs their service and commitment.

With all these and other positive attributes of the practice of medicine, what possible negativity is there that might dissuade one from its pursuit? What is there about the medical fields that could possibly negate the profession?

I'll begin with a discussion of the structural elements of medicine, some of which I've either witnessed or been a part of during my career. After that, using my protagonist Nolan as my foil, I will lay out how and why an idealistic young physician might stray.

Physicians by nature are independent-minded; usually strongwilled; and determined to call their own shots, rather than be at the mercy of others' decisions. For most physicians in the United States during the nineteenth and twentieth centuries, this meant private practice—an office that was usually owned (or leased) by the physician, who hired his own staff, which performed the myriad tasks required to run a practice. (My use of the pronoun *his,* rather than *his or hers* is intentional. There are two reasons for that: (1) Until the late twentieth century, the vast majority of physicians were male. Most medical schools either discouraged or certainly didn't go out of their way to admit women into medical school. (2) Society as well did little to encourage women to enter medicine. Rather, nursing, a perfectly admirable profession, served as the ultimate role for women. Many of these women would have performed at least as well as physicians as did the men who took up most of the medical school slots until the recent millennium.)

This has changed dramatically over the recent decades. Women now comprise the *majority* of medical school students and are rapidly increasing as a percentage of the total of all practicing physicians. My use of the masculine pronoun, therefore, is purely practical and nongender.

During the early twentieth century, medical societies began to appear. There were many reasons for that—scientific collaboration and idea sharing, social gathering of like-minded professionals the most significant of them. But in particular, it happened as physicians began to realize they would need to organize themselves if they were to become, and later on remain, an economic force in society. Hospitals were becoming powerful themselves—the Mayo and Cleveland Clinics, the Harvard-affiliated hospitals, Johns Hopkins, and other elite medical centers were influencing how medicine was practiced and delivered throughout the country. Insurance companies were beginning to dictate what methods of practice would be compensated and how much they would pay for services. Individual physicians needed an organization from which to counter the increasingly dominant forces that were determining the future of medical care.

In 1847, the American Medical Association was established. Headquartered in Chicago, it rapidly became the largest and most influential medical association in the country. State and local chapters followed, and soon, joining the AMA became a rite of passage for newly graduated physicians. The AMA developed ethical standards of practice. It established scientific organizations for virtually every field of medicine. Meetings for both education and social gathering became regular events. Specialty societies— the colleges of surgery, internal medicine, and others— were created for similar reasons. And in time, political lobbying arms were introduced so that physicians might be able to influence the myriad legislative proposals that affected virtually every aspect of medical practice, including economic issues.

I was an undergraduate student during the mid-1960s, the tumultuous time of civil rights protests and legislation, but also the Lyndon Johnson-led Medicare and Medicaid debates that ultimately led to their passage. I had heard of the AMA but, as was typical of a college student, paid it little attention. Occasionally, I read of the Medicare debates in *Newsweek* or *Time* magazines (about my only non-textbook reading sources at that time) and caught a glimpse of the process while watching a black-and-white television during *The Huntley-Brinkley Report* news hour.

Fifty-five years have dimmed my memory of the events; but I do recall hearing various physicians and politicians, including leaders of the AMA, decrying Medicare as "the first step towards socialism," maybe even communism. And some would say, or write, "This will be the death knell for the private practice of medicine." Other invectives included physicians threatening to withhold medical care from those who were enrolled in Medicare insurance.

I wondered, *Where are the doctors that supported medical care for all those in need? What happened to the voices of those who might disagree with the organized opposition to Medicare?* Well, the AMA made it quite clear that it was very strongly opposed to Medicare, Medicaid, and any other "socialized program" that would be detrimental to the interests of its members. As best I remember, there was very little organized opposition to the AMA leadership regarding those issues.

I have often wondered, over the years, what would have happened if medicine had had the equivalent of economists such as Maynard Keynes or John Kenneth Galbraith to help guide its practitioners through the legislative morass? Enlightened economists might have convinced physicians that, instead of merely opposing the proposed legislation, it would be in their interest to suggest modifications and then support the implementation of Medicare and Medicaid. That would have given physicians the opportunity to tailor these programs to suit the needs of both the public and the medical community. Naive? Maybe, but not necessarily. Perfectly designed and implemented? Almost certainly not. But better than the resultant legislation that, though providing care and economic assistance for seniors and the indigent population, contains grievous errors and inconsistencies relating to physician reimbursement.

Almost certainly, physicians would have gotten some of what they would have asked to be included in such legislation. But that was not to be the case. The AMA and its political allies stonewalled the entire process and ended up on the losing side. Medicare and Medicaid, and "Obamacare," which followed, have become staples for the provision of medical care in our country and will only increase in scope in the future. I predict that, though likely not in my lifetime, a national health system modeled after Medicare will be adopted in the United States.

When I was a medical student and later a practicing physician, I was strongly encouraged initially to join the student division and later the mainstream branch of the AMA. I, like a large percentage of my classmates and medical colleagues, declined to do so. This was because of the distaste that had developed in my mind over the AMA's complete disregard for the underserved and poorer populations of my country. Although I have been, over the years, an active participant and even an office holder in local and statewide medical associations (even serving as president of the California Radiological Society), I never joined the AMA. Rather, I continued to lobby against its positions on medical insurance for years. I listened to and occasionally verbally battled with physicians in the doctors' dining rooms and at social gatherings. Many did not agree with my positions on how to best provide medical care for everyone. I've never regretted those positions.

An analysis and thorough discussion of the high costs of medical care in the United States is beyond the scope of this book. Suffice it to say, the costs of such care is significantly higher in the United States than in all other first-world countries.6 There are no easy answers to this financial imbroglio, but failure to acknowledge, much less deal with, those costs would arguably be detrimental to our society in the future.

I chose to deal with two small segments of this dilemma by focusing on (1) the high costs of care resulting from doctor-owned surgical and imaging centers and (2) the costs resulting from physician self-referral of patients to their own facilities.

Dr. Nolan Burkett, the protagonist of my novel, becomes involved in the increasingly financially attentive world of medicine, almost without realizing what is happening. His acceptance of a role in the development of the surgicenter is the ultimate migration away from the concept of medical care for all who are in need and into the world of financial gain as a major goal for many physicians. I know this to be true because I've been there myself. In the 1980s, I was part of an unsuccessful venture for the development of an independent imaging center. And in later years, I was a partner in one that became financially very successful. Although the services provided were very good to excellent, and the physicians and staff were dedicated providers of those services, the overwhelming concern for the center was always financial. What would be good for the center and its investors? The so-called "bottom line."

Do independent centers have anything to offer patients that cannot be gained in the more traditional facilities (hospitals, private practices)? The answer is yes, especially with regard to convenience and efficiency. Hospitals are notoriously inconvenient and slowly responsive to individual patient needs. As most of us know from visits to hospital emergency rooms, for instance, wait times are often ridiculous. But I do not believe that this is enough to overcome the negatives associated with those alternative for-profit facilities. The negatives are primarily the result of self-referral, the inevitable tendency of physicians and other investors to order and perform more tests and procedures in order to generate income. Are most or all of these tests unnecessary for the patients' well-being? Of course not. But the costs are usually higher. I earlier cited two independent studies that have shown that substantially higher financial costs result more from the self-referral of services to an investor-owned medical facility than to those that are independent or publicly owned. That was certainly evident to me in my own practice and in discussions with many of my physician colleagues and friends who were similarly involved.

Another area of concern in regard to the practice of medicine in the United States is malpractice insurance.

This is another very complex situation that is well beyond the scope of this book. And I would submit that physicians are the minor rather than the major drivers of this problem. Trial lawyers have driven the costs of malpractice insurance through the proverbial roof for decades. And the public has bought into the concept that, if something has gone wrong with their or their family's care, there must be someone at fault.

Malpractice and malfeasance have occurred and will continue to do so. There are incompetent physicians, just as there are incompetent lawyers, politicians, and plumbers. Persons injured as a result of malpractice deserve financial compensation, at the very least for the direct and indirect costs resulting from errors of judgment and commission.

Relying on my own years of practice, I often heard a physician say, "I had to order that [possibly unnecessary] head CT or ultrasound exam because, if I didn't and something went wrong, I'd be sued." Yes, lawsuits can occur, on occasion. But I have always maintained— and will go to my grave doing so—that the best physicians practice medicine with little concern for malpractice. I have personally known many of them. Those competent and caring physicians believe that, if they make decisions for their patients based on sound training and medical evidence, they will not become embroiled in legal entanglement, much less incur an adverse judgement. The fact is, almost every physician has been or will be involved in a malpractice lawsuit during his or her career. But studies have proven beyond a doubt that the *overwhelming* result of lawsuits result in dismissal. By far, only the truly egregious errors result in adverse outcomes and resultant financial penalties for hospitals or physicians.

A final opinion in regard to malpractice: We, the public, as consumers, would be best served by having an independent arbitration board that is responsible for both the evaluation of and compensation for malfeasance as a result of negligence. I believe such a system could be designed with safeguards, including the right of legal appeal for all parties to a lawsuit. Such a system would not only reduce the direct and indirect costs related to medical malpractice but also arguably shorten the time between the initial event and its final disposition (which currently often stretches out for years), including prompt payment to the aggrieved.

Dr. Nolan Burkett is not unique among physicians (or people in other fields of endeavor, such as education, law, business, and a host of blue-collar positions as well). Many find themselves, for a variety of reasons, straying from their original goals and aspirations. Many continue on a straight course for the entirety of their careers, without any significant problems or incidents. In Nolan's particular case, some of his difficulties were self-inflicted, in particular those involving his marriage to Sarah. Would his marriage have suffered the same unfortunate consequences if he had continued with his surgical practice as he had originally planned? Or if he had resisted temptation from an opportunistic nurse who obviously recognized his roving eye? I chose to not explore those possibilities because I wished to explore the darker side of decision-making processes for some physicians—what may happen to those who depart from their original ideals and goals and lose sight of what attracted them to medicine in the first place.

Nolan survived, in part, because he seemed to have recognized his errors and began to make amends and to modify his behavior and how he chose to practice medicine in the future. But in the meantime, he lost his marriage, he was in danger of losing his connection with his son, and he had no idea where his relationship with Debbie would lead.

As to his professional career, we will never know whether his foray into an altruistic but unproven and professionally risky practice of medicine in a free clinic succeeds. But at least he is making the attempt. Any one of us who has been in similar situations and who has faced similar dilemmas can and should be able to relate to that.

Endnotes

1 Author's note: It is not unusual for a medical student to "dismiss" a career in a given area such as orthopedics based on limited experience with the discipline. This is particularly true during the early clinical rotation schedule, when the student is just learning the ropes and is at a decided disadvantage. The answer to this problem would be to repeat student rotations so that they could evaluate the specialty during various stages of their training.

2 Author's note: Incredibly and purely by coincidence, as I write this section of the novel, the current COVID pandemic is ravaging not only the United States but also the entire world. Having served during the AIDS epidemic, I can't help but wonder and attempt to visualize what it must be like for medical staff, as well as medical and nursing students, to attend to the needs of their patients, many of whom will succumb to this horrible affliction. The fact that the coronavirus has many of the same structural elements as the AIDS virus is both remarkable and chilling.

3 The author has noticed during his many years in medical practice that not only surgeons, but also many other physicians, are ill-prepared and/or illequipped to attend to the emotional needs of their patients and their families. Utilizing a unit of personnel including nurses, social workers, and postsurgical recovery attendants

can alleviate some of the anxiety and fear associated with surgery.

4 Author's note: Self-referral, simply put from the medical aspect, means sending (referring) a patient for an examination to a facility in which physicians (often including the one making the referral) have a financial interest. By way of example, if a cardiologist wants his or her patient to have a nuclear medicine cardiac stress test, and the study is performed either in that same office or a facility in which the cardiologist is an investor, that qualifies as a form of self-referral. It makes no difference whether the study is in the patient's best interest; often it is. But the referral benefits the referring physician financially and puts him or her in a compromised position. Is this exam truly indicated, or is it mostly just good for the economic "bottom line"?

5 Gazelle, G.S., Halpern, E.F., Ryan, H.S. "Utilization of Diagnostic Medical Imaging: Comparison of Radiologist Referral versus Same-Specialty Referral" *Radiology* 245, no. 2: 512–22; "Kickback and Physician Self-Referral," US Department of Health and Human Services.

6 News Release: Spending Highest among Developed Countries," jhsph.edu, January 7, 2019.